HIGH-T:

A Man's Guide for Boosting Testosterone

Kevin Agorastos

Copyright © 2020 Kevin Agorastos All rights reserved

The characters and events portrayed in this book are fictitious. Any similarity to real persons, living or dead, is coincidental and not intended by the author.

No part of this book may be reproduced, or stored in a retrieval system, or transmitted in any form or by any means, electronic, mechanical, photocopying, recording, or otherwise, without express written permission of the publisher.

Printed in the United States of America

Table of Contents

INTRODUCTION 1
DEFINITION OF TERMS 6
DIET AND NUTRITION 8
    Keep It Simple Stupid 8
    Read Food Labels 9
    Intermittent Fasting 11
    Macronutrients 13
    Avoid Perfection 17
10 HIGH T FOODS 18
    High T Food List 23
10 LOW T FOODS 24
PHYSICAL ACTIVITY 33
    Weight Lifting 33
    High Intensity Interval Training 35
VITAMINS AND MINERALS 38
HERBS AND SUPPLEMENTS 43
    Supplements That Probably Don't Work 47
TIPS FOR BETTER SLEEP 51
STRESS MANAGEMENT 58
    Relaxation Methods 59
    Anti-Stress Vitamins & Minerals 61
    Anti-Stress Supplements 63
    Anti-Stress Food List 64

7 SURPRISING THINGS THAT EFFECT TESTOSTERONE 65
   Plastic Containers 65
   Environmental Factors 66
   Truffle Aromatherapy 67
   Abstinence 68
   Liver Health 68
   Watching Sports 69
   Ambient Light 70

INTRODUCTION

In today's world testosterone is decreasing at an alarming rate. A 30-year-old man today has, on average, lower testosterone than his grandfather had at his age. Fifty years of research has shown that sperm quality, which correlates with testosterone levels, decreased from 113 x 10(6)/ml in 1940 to 66 x 10(6)/ml in 1990[1] Something is seriously wrong. We live in an age of unparalleled knowledge about health, diet, and physiology, yet testosterone levels are plummeting in the industrialized world. Why is this happening?

There's a variety of reasons that explains this descent including sedentary lifestyles, increased environmental toxins, and nutrient-depleted soil. Diet alone has changed dramatically in the past seven decades. Westerners typically eat a steady diet of processed foods and sugary snacks. It's a far cry from the whole natural foods our ancestors ate. Before we offer any solutions let us first look at exactly what testosterone is and what it does.

Testosterone (hence T) is the primary sex hormone in men. It's the hormone that gives men their deep voices, facial hair, broad shoulders, chiseled jawline, and sex drive. In essence, it's what makes a man a man. As a man maintaining your T levels should be a top priority. Having optimal T levels will help you to build muscle, stay lean, and live a more satisfied and fulfilled life. The consensus is that T typically peaks in the late teens and early 20s. By age 30 T starts to decline by an average of 1.25% per year. A man at age 50 will have roughly half the amount of T he had when he was in his prime. Symptoms of low T can include the following:

- Decreased sex drive
- Erectile dysfunction
- Always feeling tired (fatigue)
- Loss of vitality
- Weight gain (obesity)
- Affected memory
- Loss of lean muscle mass
- Depression and anxiety
- Irritability, moodiness
- Low self-esteem
- Hair loss
- Weaker bones
- Heart disease
- Sleep disturbances

Conventional wisdom tells us that decreased T is inevitable as men get older, or is it? Researcher David Handelsman MD, PhD, director of the ANZAC Research Institute at the University of Sydney, and his team looked at 325 men, ranging from 40 to 97 years old. All were healthy men with an average body mass index (BMI) of 26. A BMI of 25 or lower is considered healthy. Researchers then took nine separate blood samples over a 3-month period and concluded that not only did their T levels not drop but their levels did not differ despite their ages. Handelsman said "Age alone does not make you testosterone deficient... by itself, age does not cause a lower testosterone in healthy men." The keyword being "healthy". Handelsman contributes lower T to illnesses men acquire as they get older, such as cardiovascular disease and obesity. Even Handelsman's critics agree that "healthy men can have sustainable testosterone levels."[2]

Other studies support Handelsman's research. Dr. Gary Wittert, professor of medicine at the University of Adelaide, said, "It is critical that doctors understand that declining testosterone levels are not a natural part of aging and that they are most likely due to health-related behaviors or health status itself." Researchers analyzed T levels of 1,382 men between the ages of 35 and 80 years, with an average age of 54. These were healthy men who were not on any medications and had no preexisting health conditions. Their hormones were tested twice with a 5-year gap in between. It was discovered that the average T level fell only by an insignificant 1% a year between the first and second sampling five years later. Some of the biggest falls in T were from men who were either obese or depressed.[3]

Some have chosen to deal decreases T with Testosterone Replacement Therapy or TRT. TRT has gained a lot of popularity among men in recent years for its purported ability to restore youth by improving mood, libido, energy, and sexual performance among other things. Additionally, it's said to help build muscle and increase bone density. On the surface, TRT sounds great. However, TRT may not be ideal for everyone and it does come with a price.

What they usually don't tell you is once you're on TRT you're usually on it for life. That's because the body will stop its natural T production, which also causes the testicles to soften and shrink. In some instances, it's possible for the natural T production to return, but this isn't always the case. The longer someone is on it, the less likely their natural T production will return. Additionally, if treatment is abruptly stopped it can cause withdrawal symptoms including severe depression, irritability, and all the symptoms of low T. Only now it will be magnified since natural T production has completely shut down.

Possible side effects of TRT can include acne, hair loss, gynecomastia, and infertility for those under 45 years of age. TRT has also been linked to strokes and heart attacks. In 2014 the FDA demanded that T packaging include a warning of the risks to cardiovascular health in regards to TRT.[4] In the FDA's ruling, it concluded that the benefits and safety of TRT in men have yet to be established. Clearly, more research needs to be done to determine the long-term effects of TRT.

Doctors are often more than eager to put someone on TRT because they gain a customer for life. In some instances, they don't even give a blood test first or tell the patient about the potential drawbacks of TRT. Nor do they tell their patients about how lifestyle factors affect T levels. Clinical hypogonadism (failure of the testes to produce T and or sperm) is the only FDA-approved indication for TRT in men, and that it is not approved to treat age-related low T.

If you're concerned that you have low T then get your levels checked first. There are even at-home test kits you can use without going to the doctor. If test results reveal you have low T, try following the suggestions outlined in this book first. After trying all avenues and your T is still low then you might consider trying TRT. However, do your own research on the pros and cons of TRT before diving in headfirst.

The truth is most low T in men today can be attributed to poor lifestyle choices. The fix is relatively easy and a lot less expensive than TRT. What has been learned from the field of epigenetics is that we are not slaves to our genes. Our lifestyle choices, even how we think about things, can play a huge role in our health and wellbeing. That means you can maintain and even boost T levels at any age. Achieving that goal is what this book is all about. The information provided here will put you on the path to higher T, a better sex life, and a happier healthier you.

High T was written for men like you who care about their health and want to live life to the fullest at any age. The tips and suggestions offered in this book will save you time and energy of having to do all the research on your own. The information is provided in an easy-to-read format so as to not bog you down with a lot of unnecessary information and jargon. When possible, human studies are preferred over animal studies in order to provide you with the most accurate and reliable information possible.

NOTICE: The information presented in this book is intended for educational purposes only. It's not meant to replace professional medical advice. The author takes no responsibility for any damages incurred. When in doubt about something consult with your doctor first and do your own research.

DEFINITION OF TERMS

Albumin-Bound Testosterone: Albumin is a protein produced by the liver that binds with T making it unavailable for use, similar to SHBG. However, unlike SHBG the bind is weak and it can be broken and converted back into free T. Around 20% to 40% of T is albumin-bound.

Androgen: Any group of steroid hormones responsible for the development of male secondary characteristics and regulating the reproductive system. T is the most prominent and active androgen.

Aromatase: An enzyme involved in the conversion of androgen, such as T, into estrogen.

Bioavailable: The amount of a substance that is available for the body to absorb.

Cortisol: One of the primary hormones released when under stress, also known as the fight-or-flight hormone.

Dehydroepiandrosterone (DHEAS): Naturally occurring steroid hormones that act as a precursor for sex hormones, including T and estrogen.

Dihydrotestosterone (DHT): A sex steroid hormone created from T in the body. It plays a role in the development of masculine characteristics. It's considered the big brother of T.

Estrogen: The primary female sex hormone responsible for secondary sex characteristics and regulating the reproductive system. Other estrogen hormones include estrone, estradiol, and estriol.

Free Testosterone: The amount of unbound T that is available for the body to use. Typically, only 2% to 3% of total T is free T.

Human Growth Hormone (HGH): Hormone produced by the pituitary gland that plays a role in growth, cell repair, body composition, and metabolism. HGH is important for muscle growth, strength, performance, and repair.

Lignans: A type of phytoestrogen found in plant-based foods that have estrogenic properties.

Nitric Oxide (NO): A compound in the body that causes blood vessels to dilate, stimulates the release of certain hormones, and increases blood flow and oxygen levels in general.

Phytoestrogen: Naturally occurring plant nutrient that exerts an estrogenic effect on the body.

Sex Hormone-Binding Globulin (SHBG): SHBG is a protein produced by the liver and attaches to sex hormones making it unavailable for use by the body. SHBG is useful in regulating sex hormone levels. Anywhere from 60% to 80% of total T is bound to SHBG.

Total Testosterone: Also called circulating T and serum T is the total T in the body, both bound and free.

DIET AND NUTRITION

Diet and nutrition play a huge role in determining where your T levels end up. The old adage you are what you eat is very much true. You can't expect high T levels if you're on a steady diet of pizza and beer. The goal is to eat a healthy well-balanced diet consisting primarily of whole natural foods. By now most people generally know what they should and should not eat. However, a few basic dietary guidelines are in order. Don't worry, we'll get to the good stuff soon enough.

Keep It Simple Stupid

No, I'm not calling you stupid. I'm referring to the KISS principle which states things work best when kept simple. When it comes to fueling your T it's not necessary to make it more complicated than it needs to be. The main objective is to eat clean and stay away from junk foods. You probably already have a good idea of what junk foods are, so we're not going to spend a whole lot of time going into that. Just stick to the basics: stay away from soft drinks, sugary snacks, fried foods, and processed foods.

Processed foods in particular are the bane of the Western diet and are causing T levels to take a nosedive. Processed foods often contain high amounts of additives, preservatives, sugars, bad cholesterol, and bad fats. All the things that are detrimental to T levels and to health in general. For instance, a study of 209 men demonstrated that those who consumed high amounts of trans-fat had a 15% decrease in T levels and a 37% lower sperm count from those who consumed lower amounts of it.[5]

Instead, eat a diet consisting of lean meats, copious amounts of vegetables, and a moderate amount of fruits. You want to focus on eating whole foods that are preferably organic. Organic foods will admittedly cost you more, but it's worth it to your health and T levels in the long run. Non-organic foods are prone to environmental toxins from pesticides which negatively affect T levels and are bad for your overall health in general. We will get into the specifics of what to eat and what not to eat shortly.

Read Food Labels

Part of being healthy is taking responsibility for what you are eating. When you're at the store always read the food labels and pay close attention to the ingredients. Even so-called healthy foods may contain ingredients that are anything but healthy. Here are some helpful tips to keep in mind when reading food labels:

- ❖ Natural is always better. If you're reading a food label and you see an ingredient you can't pronounce then odds are good it's not natural. Try to avoid foods with additives and preservatives. They are nothing more than harmful man-made chemicals.

❖ Ingredients are arranged on a food label in order of quantity, from greatest to least. This is a good indicator of how much each ingredient is in what you're eating. When it comes to ingredients less is often more. A good food option is one with the least amount of ingredients.

❖ Stay away from artificial sweeteners. They are often just as bad if not worse than refined sugar. Artificial sugars include aspartame, NutraSweet, Splenda, sorbitol, and Sweet 'N Low among many others. Better natural sweeteners are stevia, coconut sugar, fruit purees, maple syrup, and raw honey.

❖ Salt is sometimes disguised under different names such as sodium, monosodium glutamate (MSG), and disodium guanylate (GMP). Ideally, keep your salt intake to around 480 mg or less and do not exceed more than 1,000 mg per day.

❖ Avoid products that include "partially hydrogenated" in the list of ingredients. Partially hydrogenated is a code word for trans-fat which clogs arteries, raises bad cholesterol, and lowers T levels. The FDA does not require manufacturers to list trans-fat if it's less than 0.5 g. That means a product with 0.4 g of trans-fat could be labeled as "trans-fat free" or "zero trans-fat". That's why it's always important to read the label. Fully hydrogenated products do not contain trans-fat so they are not as bad as partially hydrogenated products. However, that doesn't mean they're necessarily healthier either.

❖ Pay attention to the serving size. The calories and nutrients listed on the food label are in relation to the serving size. For instance, if one serving is listed on the label and you eat two servings, then you're consuming double the calories and double the nutrients listed on the food label.

❖ Sucrose, glucose, high fructose corn syrup, maple syrup, and fructose are all sugars. The American Heart Association recommends that men should consume no more than 38 g of sugar daily. However, less is definitely more when it comes to sugar intake.

Intermittent Fasting

Perhaps you may have already heard about intermittent fasting (IF). IF is simply the process of limiting the eating window to a shorter timeframe. Everyone fasts while they're asleep. Typically, IF just extends that fasting period until later in the day. IF has gained a lot of popularity in recent years and for good reason. The benefits of IF are numerous and includes the following:

➢ Promotes weight loss by consuming fewer calories

➢ Promotes longevity by inducing cellular repair and altering gene expression in positive ways

➢ Promotes healthy brain function and wards off degenerative neurological diseases

➢ Reduces Inflammation and oxidative stress

> Improves blood sugar by reducing insulin levels, which helps reverse type 2 diabetes

> Keeps the heart healthy by increasing good HDL cholesterol and reducing bad LDL cholesterol

> Increases human growth hormone by as much as 5-fold, which facilitates fat burning and muscle growth

In regards to T, IF is beneficial in two ways. First, whenever you eat your glucose levels automatically rise. This is especially true when you eat carbs or sugars. As a result, your pancreas will produce insulin to transport the glucose from your bloodstream into your cells so it can be converted into energy. However, if your insulin is too high for too long and too often, it can eventually lead to insulin resistance, which can cause type 2 diabetes. High insulin is linked to decreased T levels.

In one study, 74 men were given a standard dose of 75 g of pure glucose to determine the effects of glucose on T. Researchers discovered that the glucose solution decreased blood levels of T by as much as 25%. It didn't matter if the men had diabetes, prediabetes, or a normal glucose tolerance. Even after two hours, 73 of the 74 men continued to show reduced T levels. IF solves the problem of insulin spikes simply by eating less often.[6]

Second, IF has been shown to increase T by as much as 180%.[7] One of the ways it does this is by increasing growth hormone levels, which correlates with higher T levels. A study done at the University of Virginia Medical School showed that not eating for 24 hours led to a threefold increase in growth hormone levels.[8] This makes it especially beneficial for weightlifters.

One of the most common types of IF is 16:8 fasting. This means that in a 24-hour period you have an 8-hour eating window. For many that will involve skipping breakfast and eating a late lunch. Of course, this may not be ideal for everyone's schedule. The great thing about IF is that it's highly customizable. You can arrange your eating window to include breakfast or however you would like. Personally, I don't follow a strict eating window. Just do whatever works best for your lifestyle and schedule.

If you're not used to IF it may take a little time for your body to adjust. At first, it might seem difficult and you may even feel fatigued, but your body will soon adapt. I like to work out while in a fasted state, but if you've never tried IF before then I recommend not to work out fasted until your body has had time to adjust to it. Otherwise, your energy levels may be low and your workouts will be a struggle.

Macronutrients

Macros are short for macronutrients and they include proteins, carbohydrates (carbs), and fats. Having a proper ratio is important for maximizing weight loss, muscle gain, and optimizing T. Your needs will vary depending on your age, weight, height, job, and goals. If you're trying to gain muscle then your macros should be 20% fat, 35% protein, and 45% carbs. If you're trying to lose weight your target macros should be 20% to 35% fat, 35% to 50% protein, and 25% to 45% carbs. And if you're in maintenance mode your macros should be 25% to 40% fat, 25% to 40% protein, and 35% to 55% carbs.

Protein: Protein sources come in two varieties, animal and vegetable. Animal protein includes lean beef (preferably grass-fed), chicken, fish (in moderation), and turkey. Vegetable protein options include lentils, nuts, seeds, and beans, just to name a few. It's necessary to get adequate amounts of protein in your diet. Diets low in protein have been shown to increase SHBG and decrease T bioactivity.[9] The reason for this is because if SHBG levels are too high it binds to T leaving less free T readily available in the bloodstream. The more free T you have available the better.

There is much debate regarding rather animal or protein is superior for T production. The studies don't seem to be much help either. For every study that shows animal protein is superior for T production another study will say the exact opposite. So, which is better, animal or vegetable protein?

I generally side with animal protein for the main reason that it contains the necessary fats required for T production. On the other hand, dietary fats from vegetables are generally low. Vegetarians and vegans consume lower levels of saturated fats than omnivores. Furthermore, the fats obtained through vegetables are mostly polyunsaturated fatty acids (PUFA), which lowers T production. As a result, vegan diets can lead to lower levels of total and free T with higher levels of SHBG.

To illustrate this point, a study involving 43 healthy men, aged 19 to 56, were assigned to either a low-fat, high-fiber diet or a high-fat, low-fiber diet for 10 weeks. The mean plasma concentrations of total T and SHBG bound T was 13% to 15% higher for those on the high-fat, low-fiber diet. Their daily urinary excretion of T also was 13% higher with the high-fat, low-fiber diet than with the low-fat, high-fiber diet.[10]

As an added bonus, there is also a correlation between strength training while on a diet of higher healthy fats and T levels. A study of 8 strength athletes and 10 physically active non-athletes demonstrated that heavy resistance training, specifically high volume and high intensity, in conjunction with a diet of fats and protein was directly correlated with serum T and free T levels.[11]

Lastly, animal protein has nutrients that are either very difficult or impossible to get from plants alone including vitamin B12, creatine, carnosine, vitamin D3, DHA, iron, and taurine. As with all things, anything can be overdone. Animal protein should be eaten as part of a balanced diet.

Carbohydrates: Carbs are our primary source of energy. They often get a bad rap, but they're important to our health and wellbeing. Without them we would be fatigued all the time, not to mention irritable. While carbs are good too much can cause you to gain weight, especially the wrong kind of carbs.

There are two types of carbs: simple and complex carbs. Simple carbs break down quickly when digested causing a spike in blood glucose, often called a sugar rush. Candy, sugary snacks, soda, milk, white pasta and bread are all examples of simple carbs. Generally, you'll want to stay away from simple carbs, although not all simple carbs are bad. Some fruit and vegetables are also simple carbs. However, because they are nutrient-dense and fibrous they help to balance things out and should be included in everyone's diet. Although it's still best to eat fruits in moderation.

Complex carbs, on the other hand, break down more slowly making them the preferred carbohydrate. Complex carbs can be found in nuts, beans, whole grains, fruits, and some vegetables. When it comes to things like bread, pasta, and rice the general rule of thumb is the darker the better. So, whole-grain bread, brown rice, and whole-grain pasta are better options than white bread, white rice, and white pasta. Carb intake should ideally be a little higher on days you work out and a little lower on rest days, or days when energy consumption is not very high.

Fats: Contrary to popular belief, not all fats are bad. Healthy fats are in fact essential in order to maintain healthy T levels. A study conducted by the *Journal of Steroid Biochemistry* concluded that a decrease in dietary fats coincided with a decrease in total T and free T.[12] Other studies have confirmed that low-fat high-fiber diets resulted in a 12% lowering of circulating androgen levels. Androgens are the hormones responsible for male characteristics and reproduction.[13] Needless to say, T production is heavily dependent upon dietary fat intake. A diet with less than 20% of your calories from fat will limit your body's production of T.

There are three types of fat we want to focus on. The first is saturated fat, which is found in foods such as red meat, egg yolks, coconut oil, and fermented dairy products like goat's milk, kefir, yogurt, and goat cheese. People don't usually think of saturated fat as being healthy because it's purportedly linked with high cholesterol levels and heart disease. However, additional research is showing that processed fats such as trans-fats and hydrogenated fats are more likely the culprit. Saturated fats in the right amounts can be healthy and are crucial for optimal T levels.

The second source of fats is polyunsaturated fats which include omega-3 fatty acids and omega-6 fatty acids. Polyunsaturated fats can be found in seafood such as salmon, mackerel, herring, sardines, etc. Be aware that certain types of fish can contain high levels of mercury. You may wish to consider limiting your seafood consumption and get your omega-3s primarily from fish oil supplements. Polyunsaturated fats can also be found in chia seeds and walnuts. We need both omega-3 and omega-6 in our diet, but too much omega-6 can be detrimental to T levels.

The third fat is monounsaturated fats which are a type of unsaturated fat. Monounsaturated fats are healthy fats found in avocados, almonds, peanut butter, and oils such as olive, canola, safflower, sesame, and peanut oil. Olive oil is an especially good monounsaturated fat. Participants who consumed extra-virgin olive oil over a three-week period increased their T levels by 17 to 19 percent.[14]

Avoid Perfection

While the goal is to eat healthy the majority of the time, no diet will be sustainable if it's too strict. There has to be some flexibility built-in if it's to be maintained for the long term. A good rule to follow is the 80/20 rule. That means you should strive to eat healthy 80 percent of the time, and eat what you want the rest of the 20 percent. The 80/20 rule is a daily rule to follow. However, you can set aside one cheat day every week or better yet one cheat meal a week. You only live once, so don't feel guilty about indulging once in a while.

10 HIGH T FOODS

There are many great foods that will aid you in your quest for optimal T. To list each one would fill an entire book in itself. Instead, we're going to focus on 10 of the most commonly listed high T foods.

1. Cruciferous Vegetables: Remember when you were told as a kid to eat your veggies? Well, as it turns out they were right. Cruciferous vegetables are great anti-estrogenic foods. Cruciferous vegetables are part of the Brassicaceae family and includes broccoli, cabbage, cauliflower, kale, and Brussels sprouts. These vegetables contain a nutrient called indole-3-carbinol (I-3-C) and coverts to diindolylmethane (DIM) in the stomach to help cleanse the body of excess estrogen. DIM is also available in supplement form. As an added benefit, cruciferous vegetables may help reduce the risk of certain cancers, protect the body against harmful radiation, and rid the body of harmful toxins.

2. Eggs: Eggs have been the topic of considerable debate due to their high cholesterol content. For decades during the 1970s and 1980s, the public was advised not to eat eggs. That began to change in 1999 when a leading medical journal found no link between eggs and cardiovascular disease.[15] As it turns out, cholesterol is a necessary precursor for all sex hormones, including T. Eggs are also a great source of protein, vitamin D, and omega-3s, which aid in the production of T. It's safe to eat up to three eggs daily which raises the HDL "good" cholesterol.[16] Studies have noted the relationship between increased HDL cholesterol and increased free T.[17] Additional high cholesterol foods include organ meats, shellfish, and full-fat cheese.

3. Mushrooms: Mushrooms are a type of fungus that is packed with protein, vitamins, minerals, and antioxidants. There are many varieties of mushrooms including Portobello, shiitake, chanterelle, and white button mushrooms. Not a whole lot of research has been done on mushrooms in regards to T, but there is some evidence to suggest white button mushrooms, in particular, have anti-estrogenic properties.[18] This is accomplished by suppressing aromatase activity, which is an enzyme that's responsible for estrogen production.

4. Raw Cacao: Raw cacao is a type of unheated minimally processed chocolate that has numerous health benefits and is loaded with antioxidants, minerals, and healthy fats. Cacao contains the highest source of flavonols, which are known to increase nitric oxide concentrations and bioavailability. Additionally, these antioxidants help reduce stress and cortisol levels. Reducing stress is so important for optimizing T levels that a whole chapter has been devoted to it.

Raw cacao contains many of the minerals necessary for T production including zinc, magnesium, calcium, iron, and manganese, just to name a few. One 35-gram bar alone can provide 20% of the daily recommend allowance of zinc. Last but not least, raw cacao helps to regulate blood sugar and lower bad cholesterol, all of which impact T levels. This makes raw cacao a great well-rounded snack to include in your diet.

5. Honey: Honey is an all-around great T booster. It contains vitamin B, protein, magnesium, as well as the trace mineral boron. Aside from helping to build muscle and bone, boron has been shown to beneficially impact the body's use of estrogen, T, and vitamin D.[19] Darker honey is preferred as it has higher concentrations of minerals over lighter honey. That's not all, just three-ounces of honey has been shown to increase nitric oxide levels in the bloodstream, which leads to better blood flow, circulation, and oxygen in the body. For men, that also means better sexual function.

6. Bananas: Aside from being a great snack, bananas are known to boost energy, increase libido, and raise T levels. Bananas contain an enzyme called bromelain that is important in the production of T. In fact, cyclists who were given bromelain were able to maintain their concentration of T over a six-day cycle stage race.[20] Bananas also contain a lot of great minerals for T production including vitamin B6 and magnesium. B6 is one of the best types of B vitamins for T optimization. What's more, bananas contain vitamin C which has been shown to reduce the stress hormone cortisol. Bananas are high in sugar so eat them in moderation and while they are still partially ripe.

7. Raisins: Raisins are a great snack that's packed with the antioxidant resveratrol. Resveratrol is a compound commonly found in the skin of grapes. Some studies have indicated resveratrol acts as an inhibiter to estrogen synthesis.[21] Resveratrol has additional cardiovascular benefits and can improve nitric oxide availability. Raisins contain the densest source of boron, which as previously noted is linked to higher T levels. Just 100 mg of raisins contain 100% of the recommended daily allowance of boron.

8. Wild Salmon: There's a lot to like when it comes to salmon. For starters, it's packed with all the key vitamins and minerals necessary for optimal T production: vitamin B, vitamin D, zinc, and magnesium. Salmon is also a great source of omega-3 fatty acids. These fatty acids increase the levels of luteinizing hormone to raise T production while lowering SHBG levels. Less SHBG means more available free T.

Wild salmon is preferred over farm-raised salmon as it contains higher levels of nutrients compared to its farm-raised counterpart. Additionally, farmed raised salmon has been linked to higher levels of omega-6 fatty acids and higher levels of contaminants. Still, even wild salmon should be eaten in moderation. Limit your intake of wild salmon to no more than two to three severing a week at most.

9. Oysters: If you love oysters then you're in luck. Oysters are a great T boosting super-food. In addition to being an excellent source of protein, they contain all the best vitamins and minerals for T production including magnesium, vitamin D, and zinc. Oysters contain almost seven times the recommended daily allowance of zinc. What's more, oysters are an excellent source of omega-3 fatty acids.

Oysters contain an amino acid called D-aspartic acid (DAA) that acts as a precursor to T production. In some studies, DAA showed a significant increase in T levels by as much as 42%.[22] Although not all studies indicate that DAA is beneficial, more on that later.

There's one more good reason to eat oysters. They've been known as an aphrodisiac as far back as ancient Rome. There's a reason why the notorious ladies' man Giacomo Casanova was said to have eaten 50 oysters for breakfast every day!

10. **Pumpkin Seeds:** Pumpkin seeds are a great antioxidant snack that's rich in iron, zinc, magnesium, healthy fats, and other valuable nutrients, all of which play a role in maintaining healthy T levels. What's more, they are one of the best sources of magnesium available. Pumpkin seeds also contain an amino acid called leucine. Leucine supplementation was studied in male athletes.[23] It was observed that leucine increased serum T levels by as much as 20% during a 5-week period.

BONUS

Avocados: Avocados are one of the best non-meat sources of the healthy fats needed for good T levels. One whole avocado contains 4.2g of saturated fat, nearly 20g of monounsaturated fat, and 3.6g of polyunsaturated fat. It's packed full of vitamins and minerals including magnesium, potassium, vitamin C, vitamin E, zinc, niacin (vitamin B3), vitamin K, iron, and copper. If you're taking a lot of zinc, you'll want to eat avocados as zinc can deplete copper levels. Avocados can additionally improve heart health, lower bad cholesterol, and reduce inflammation. Best of all they contain less than 1g of sugar.

High T Food List

There are many food options available that will help to boost and optimize T levels. The following is a partial list of foods you may want to include in your diet.

Cabbage	Asparagus	Watermelon
Spinach	Shellfish	Avocados
Green Leafy Vegetables	Pineapple	Onions
Tuna	Red Grapes	Potatoes
Pomegranate	Extra-Virgin Olive Oil	Beets
Parsley	Ginger	Macadamia Nuts
Wheat Bran	Unprocessed Meats	Blue Cheese
Yogurt	Dark Berries	Coconut & Coconut Oil
Brazil Nuts	Strawberries	Sorghum
Lemons	Kiwi	Tomatoes
Red Bell Peppers	Chai Seeds	Cauliflower

10 LOW T FOODS

Sometimes it's not always about what to eat but also about what not to eat that's important. The following are 10 foods that can potentially decrease T levels and should be minimized or avoided altogether.

1. Sugar: This one really shouldn't come as a surprise. Sugar rather it's from fructose, sucrose, lactose, or glucose raises insulin, which directly correlates to lower T levels. Sugar is also linked to weight gain and obesity. Moderate obesity decreases total T due to insulin resistance and severe obesity decreases free T due to suppression of the HPT axis. This creates a vicious cycle as insulin resistance leads to lower T and lower T leads to insulin resistance. Therefore, the goal should be to minimize refined sugars as much as possible.

2. Alcohol: According to the National Survey on Drug Use and Health, 80% of people who were surveyed consumed alcohol at some point in their lives. For many, alcohol is an occasional social activity they do with friends to help them unwind. The problem is when there's an overconsumption of alcohol. Drinking 2 to 3 alcoholic drinks per day over a 3-week period can decrease T levels by nearly 7% in men.[24] Other studies have confirmed an association with acute alcohol consumption and decreased T levels in men.[25] Additionally, alcohol is linked to weight gain and other health risks. One of the worst offenders is beer. Beer contains hops, a known phytoestrogen that mimics estrogen and lowers T levels. If you're going to drink then do so in moderation.

3. Soy: The concerns over soy can best be summed up with the following story about a man named James Price. At 55 years old, retired U.S. Army Intelligence Officer James Price began to experience unusual symptoms. He started to develop breasts that were painful and swollen to the touch. His beard growth had slowed, he started losing body hair, and his sexual desire disappeared completely. Even his emotions began to change. He would cry while watching sad movies, which wasn't typical for him. For all intent and purposes his body seemed to be feminizing, but why?

Mr. Price sought the medical attention of three different doctors, all who had diagnosed him with gynecomastia or abnormal enlargement of the mammary glands in men. They also discovered he had eight times more estrogen in his bloodstream than normal, even higher than that of a healthy woman. The problem was the doctors couldn't figure out the cause of it. One of his doctors got so frustrated he even accused Mr. Price of secretly taking estrogen.

Mr. Price became frustrated but decided to try one more doctor as a last resort, a fellow military man named Lieutenant Colonel Jack E. Lewi, M.D. Dr. Lewi was chief of endocrinology at the San Antonio Military Medical Center. At first, Dr. Lewi was also stumped. Every test seemed to come back negative. Finally, Dr. Lewi began to examine Mr. Price's lifestyle habits with a little more scrutiny. What he discovered was Price had been drinking an average of 3 quarts of soy milk a day. Price had initially switched to soy milk after developing an intolerance to regular milk.

Suddenly Dr. Lewi had found the cause of Price's elevated estrogen levels. The culprit, as it turns out, was soy. After removing the soy from his diet his estrogen levels slowly began to return to normal levels after several months. However, not all of his estrogen-related symptoms completely disappeared. His loss of libido and heightened emotions persisted. And while the pain in his breasts disappeared the swelling remained.[26]

Stories such as the one involving James Price has made soy an extremely controversial topic. Detractors will say that soy lowers T in men, while proponents of soy will say it's all a myth and doesn't have any effect on T levels. So who's right? The truth lies somewhere in the middle.

Studies on soy's effect on T are admittedly mixed. One study found that 35 men who drank soy protein isolate for 54 days had decreased T levels, including a minor effect on other hormones.[27] In a Harvard study in the journal *Human Reproduction*, Jorge E. Chavarro, M.D and his colleagues found a strong association between men consuming soy and lower sperm counts.[28] However, other peer-reviewed clinical studies have concluded that "neither soy foods nor isoflavone supplements alter measures of bioavailable T concentrations in men."[29] Clearly, there's more human-based research that needs to be done.

What we do know is that soy contains a high concentration of isoflavones, specifically genistein and daidzein. Isoflavonoids and their derivatives are called phytoestrogens because they can mimic human estrogen in the body. Studies on phytoestrogens in leading peer-reviewed medical journals suggest that even at lower doses, such as the FDA's recommended 25 g of soy protein a day, can wreak havoc on hormones. For men, this can mean lower libido, weight gain, low stamina, loss of virility, and the dreaded man boobs.

James Price was likely an outlier who had an acute sensitivity to soy. He also drank way more soy than the average person. Not everyone will necessarily have the same experience as Mr. Price. Everyone is different and soy will affect everyone's hormones to different degrees as well. For some phytoestrogens may only mildly affect their hormones. Still, even a mild effect is not going to do your T levels any favors.

I would generally err on the side of caution if for no other reason than 90% of the soy in the US is genetically modified and has the highest percentage of contamination of pesticides, which adversely affect T levels. The herbicide Roundup is commonly used on GMO crops and contains the chemical compound glyphosate. A study on rat testicular cells showed that even non-toxic levels of glyphosate lowered T by 35%.[30] For this reason, soy is on the low T list.

Does that mean all soy is bad? Not necessairly. Fermented soy, such is typically eaten in Asia is acceptable. These include tempeh, natto, and miso, among others. The reason for this is soy loses a lot of its lectin, phytate, and phytoestrogen content during the fermentation process. In fact, the level of isoflavones is reduced by as much as 300% during fermentation. Westerns, on the other hand, mostly consume non-fermented soy.

In conclusion, if soy is organic and fermented then it's perfectly acceptable to eat. Otherwise, it would be best to avoid soy products for the reasons stated. If the goal is to have optimal T levels, then it's best to avoid anything which could potentially lower it, even by a marginal amount. And now you know the rest of the story.

4. **Flaxseed:** Flaxseed is chockfull of vitamins, minerals, antioxidants, omega-3 fatty acids, and is purported to have many other health benefits. Unfortunately, it contains a type of phytoestrogen called lignans, which has an estrogenic effect in the body. Flaxseed has the highest concentrations of lignans, some 74 to 800 times higher than cereal grains, legumes, fruits, and vegetables.[31] Flaxseed will also increase SHBG levels. There's admittedly not a lot of studies on the effects of lignans on males. Still, it's better to err on the side of caution and avoid flaxseed.

5. **Milk & Dairy:** In recent years there have been concerns over the hormones and steroids in cow's milk. Cow's milk is reported to contain up to 50 hormones in total including growth hormone, prolactin, glucocorticoids, androgens, and female sex hormones. This has made cow's milk somewhat controversial. Proponents argue that concerns over cow's milk are largely over-exaggerated. However, there are several studies which do confirm the concerns over cow's milk.

The milk we consume today differs greatly from the milk consumed 100 years ago. Genetically improved dairy cows continue to lactate throughout almost their entire pregnancy. As a result, cow's milk contains large amounts of estrogen and progesterone. In one small study, men who drank cow's milk had significant increases in estrone and progesterone concentrations and significant decreases in their T concentrations.[32] It's been estimated that milk and dairy products account for as much as 60% to 70% of all animal-derived estrogens consumed.[33]

In another study, data was gathered from several databases including MEDLINE, ScienceDirect, Google Scholar and Web of Science.[34] The results indicate the presence of steroid hormones in dairy products that could be counted as an important risk factor for various cancers in humans. The main estrogen in cow's milk is estradiol, followed by estrone and oestradiol. They found the maximum concentration of total estrone in butter, followed by cream, Gouda cheese, yogurt, and milk.

Organic cow's milk is not much better. While organic cow's milk may contain fewer pesticides and growth hormones, the estrogen levels can be even higher than regular cow's milk. As an alternative try goat's milk. Goat's milk has fewer toxins and lower estrogen levels than cow's milk. If you want to go a step further there are non-dairy alternatives such as almond milk, which doesn't contain any estrogens at all.

6. Licorice: You might be familiar with licorice in products such as cough mixtures, gums, teas, drinks, and candies. Licorice comes from the root of a plant that's native to Asia and Southern Europe. It may seem like an unlikely culprit, but licorice consumption has been linked with a reduction in serum T levels in healthy men. One of the main compounds in licorice, glycyrrhizic acid, inhibits an enzyme in the Leydig cells that blocks T production. This was confirmed in a study that found licorice consumption decreased T levels by as much as 26%.[35]

Licorice doesn't only lower T levels but at least one human study showed that it increases estrogen.[36] The *American Association for Cancer Research* was looking at natural compounds that would improve women's health by mimicking estrogen. Licorice root was selected because it contains the phytoestrogen glabridin whose structure resembles the female sex hormone estradiol. It was shown that glabridin did indeed produce estrogen-like activities. That's not all. It's also been found that glycyrrhetinic acid, a hydrolytic product of glycyrrhizic acid, inhibits certain enzymes resulting in increases in the stress hormone cortisol.[37] More cortisol equals lower T.

7. Nuts: People are nuts about nuts. Who can blame them? They do make great snacks. However, while nuts have health benefits there are good reasons to limit your consumption of them. For starters, some types of nuts are known to increase SHBG. In particular, walnuts by 12% and almonds by 16%.[38]

Secondly, they contain a lot of omega-6 fatty acids. Omega-6 is not bad in itself, but it must be balanced with omega-3. Otherwise, it can become unhealthy and decrease T levels. Lastly, nuts contain compounds called phytosterols. Phytosterols lower cholesterol, which as we've already established is necessarily for T production.

This doesn't mean you have to eliminate nuts completely from your diet, only that they should be eaten in moderation. You also want to focus on nuts that have more omega-3 and less omega-6. These include Brazil nuts and macadamia nuts.

8. Microwave Popcorn: Everyone loves eating popcorn on movie night, but it can also kill your T. The problem with microwave popcorn is the bags they come in are often lined with chemicals such as perfluorooctanoic acid (PFOA), which can wreak havoc on your endocrine system and T levels. In addition, PFOA has been connected with kidney cancer, testicular cancer, thyroid disease, and high cholesterol. While PFOA has been banned in the U.S., it can still be found in imported products. Theater popcorn may also contain PFOA chemicals.

PFOA has largely been replaced by GenX, but this has only replaced one chemical with another. Recent studies indicate that GenX could be a more potent liver toxin than PFOA. GenX is still fairly new and the full effects may not be known for some time. The problems don't stop with the bag lining either. The artificial butter substitute in microwave popcorn can contain a chemical called diacetyl which has been linked to a repertory disease called popcorn lung. In some instances, diacetyl has been replaced by other diacetyl substitutes, which are just as toxic.

Popcorn in itself is not bad as long as it's all-natural organic popcorn that doesn't come in a microwavable bag. Consuming popcorn can actually be good for your T levels. It contains a number of vitamins and minerals, including zinc and magnesium. We'll talk more about these minerals in a bit.

9. Legumes and beans: Legumes refer to a particular group of plants while beans are a subcategory of legumes. These include foods such as lentils, lima beans, peas, green beans, mung beans, and soybeans. Legumes and beans are sometimes considered good T foods due to their high protein and zinc content. The problem is studies have shown several legumes are also a source of phytoestrogens with high levels of estrogenic activity.[39] Some legumes and beans contain a type of phytoestrogen called coumestan. Coumestan represents less than 1% of all estrogenic foods, yet makes up 30% of the total phytoestrogen content in legumes and beans. This doesn't mean you have to remove legumes and beans completely from your diet, only limit your consumption of them.

10. Vegetable oils: Vegetable oils are oils that are liquid at room temperature and include canola, soybean, corn, peanut, and palm, safflower, and cottonseed oil. These oils can be found in everything from potato chips, margarine, baked goods, to pizzas and burgers. These are not natural oils but refined and highly processed oils using chemicals that change their makeup. These oils were not even available until the 20th century.

The problem with vegetable oils is the same as with most nuts, they are high in omega-6 polyunsaturated fatty acids. We've already established the correlation between too much omega-6 and reduced T. The Western diet contains far too much omega-6s and not enough omega-3s. Historically, the humans had a diet with a ratio of omega 6 to omega 3 of approximately 1:1 whereas the Western diet has ratios of 15/1 to 16.7/1.[40]

Refined vegetable oils can also contain trans-fat causing inflammation. Better alternatives are oils that are higher in omega-3s and are made by crushing or pressing plants and seeds. Extra-virgin olive oil, avocado oil, grapeseed oil, and coconut oil are all better options.

PHYSICAL ACTIVITY

Weight Lifting

One of the best things you can do for your T levels, besides having a good diet, is weightlifting. Weightlifting will give you an immediate short-term boost in T, albeit temporarily. The effects will subside within a few hours after working out. Nevertheless, that doesn't mean it's not beneficial. Weightlifting has been shown to increase growth hormone and T in the young and old alike.[41] The fact is men who lift weights, and keep fit in general, are going to have higher resting T rates than the guys who never hit the gym.

When training to increase T the focus should be on lifting moderate to heavy weights. Generally speaking, the heavier the better. How heavy depends upon your ability to maintain proper form while hitting your rep ranges. You don't want to lift more weight than you can handle. If you don't feel confident about lifting a certain weight, then drop it down to something more manageable. Then work to progressively increase the weight from there. Don't let your ego compel you to lift more weight than you are currently capable of. And always remember, practice good form so you don't end up injuring yourself.

The primary focus when lifting weights should be on compound movements. Compound movements involve utilizing two or more joints at the same time. For example, squats are a compound movement because it's using both the hip and knee joints. On the other hand, isolated movements utilize only one joint at a time. Curls are an example of an isolated movement because it's only utilizing the elbow joint. That doesn't mean that you shouldn't do isolated movements. Only that for boosting T, compound movements will elicit a greater effect on T levels than isolated movements. Compound movements will additionally allow you to work more than one muscle group at the same time, giving you the most bang for the buck.

When it comes to building muscle and boosting T, the primary compound lifts are squats, chin-ups\pull-ups, dips, bench press, deadlifts, shoulder overhead press, and barbell row. That's it! You could build a solid physique using only these seven exercises. Stick with free-weights rather than machine weights. A study comparing squats to the leg press showed a greater hormonal response from squatting.[42] This applies to other free-weight exercises as well.

Additionally, consider implementing reverse pyramid training. Reverse pyramid training lowers the weight after every set by 5 to 10 lbs. or as needed. For instance, on the first set lift the most weight you can. Then on the next set lower the weight by 10 lbs. and so on. This will allow you to lift the most amount of weight while also accounting for diminishing returns.

Rest periods between sets should generally be between 1 to 3 minutes, depending on the intensity of the exercise. The more intense the exercise the more time will be needed for recovery. I generally prefer 2 minutes, although research has shown short rest periods elicit a higher hormonal response. However, you don't want your rest periods to be too short either. You need to give your nervous system time to recover so you can lift the most amount of weight possible on the next set.

For the greatest hormonal response to occur you really need to push yourself. However, limit your workouts to no more than one hour. Keep in mind that working out is a form of stress, and too much exercise can start to increase cortisol levels and decrease T levels. Giving your body time to rest and recuperate is just as important as working out. Depending upon your routine you should rest at the least one day a week or more if needed. It's entirely possible to make progress working out just three times per week.

For an added boost, try taking caffeine before your workouts. T response to exercise was shown to increase with caffeine when compared against a placebo.[43] Sleep is also important. Make sure to get a good night's sleep so it doesn't negatively impact your work out performance the next day. There will be more tips on how to optimize your sleep in an upcoming chapter.

High Intensity Interval Training

Cardio is another great way to boost T levels, but it should be short and strategic. What you want to avoid is endurance-type exercises, which will only decrease T levels. Instead, focus on quick but intense cardio sessions. One way to accomplish this is with High Intensity Interval Training or HITT. HITT raises T levels by 92% compared to only 62% with low-intensity exercises.[44]

There are various types of HITT workouts, but the basic idea is to pick an exercise and do it at maximum intensity followed by brief rest periods. That cycle is repeated until the workout is complete. Some additional benefits of HITT include:

- Burns a lot of calories in a short amount of time, saving time
- Reduces heart rate and blood pressure
- Weight loss
- Raises metabolic rate for hours after exercise
- Improves oxygen consumption
- Reduces blood sugar
- Boosts human growth hormone
- Reduces the stress hormone cortisol

One popular form of HITT is Tabata training. Tabata was created by Dr. Izumi Tabata and his team of researchers. Dr. Tabata and his team researched two groups of athletes. The first group trained an hour at moderate-intensity five days a week for six weeks. The second group trained at high-intensity four days a week for six weeks.

The moderate-intensity group increased their aerobic (cardiovascular) system but showed little to no results to their anaerobic (muscular) system. The high-intensity group, on the other hand, showed not only a greater increase to their aerobic system but also increased their anaerobic system by 28%. The conclusion was sometimes less is more. The high-intensity group had a greater impact on the aerobic and anaerobic systems in less time than the moderate-intensity group.

Tabata only lasts for 4 minutes and consists of a cycle of 20 seconds of intense exercise followed by a 10 second rest period. If that sounds easy think again. Try a Tabata workout alternating between burpees and mountain climbers at maximum intensity. You'll discover that 4 minutes never felt so long.

Another way to get an intense cardio workout in a short amount of time is with plyometrics, also called jump training. Plyometrics are fast explosive movements that stimulate the fast-twitch muscle fibers. They are very fast and very dynamic movements that incorporate speed, stability, mobility, and strength. They will also wear you out quickly. Plyometric exercises include box jumps, burpees, jump squats, tuck jumps, and jump lunges. YouTube is a great resource to demonstrate these exercises and many others.

Finally, sprinting is another excellent T boosting workout. It's great for building strength, endurance, cardiovascular health, and athletic performance in general. Sprint all out for 10 to 20 seconds, take a brief rest period, and repeat 4 to 8 times. Warming up is extremely important, and if you've never sprinted before it may be necessary to work up to it.

Sprinting doesn't just apply to running, but any activity that involves performing at top speed for short intervals. Duration also matters. The HGH response was compared between the 6-second and 30-second cycle ergometer sprint. Serum HGH concentration for the 30-second sprint was 450% greater than the 6-second sprint. HGH levels continued to stay elevated for 1.5 to 2 hours after the sprint program.[45]

VITAMINS AND MINERALS

There is a multitude of vitamins and minerals on the market that come in a variety of shapes and sizes. While they all have their uses there's only a handful that have a meaningful effect on T levels. I call them the T trifecta of vitamin D, zinc, and magnesium. They will not boost your T per se but they will help to maintain optimal T levels.

Vitamin D: Vitamin D, specifically vitamin D3, plays a crucial role in T production. Men with sufficient vitamin D levels have significantly higher levels of free T and significantly lower levels of SHBG.[46] Unfortunately, most people are deficient in vitamin D. In the United States alone nearly half the population is deficient in vitamin D, and even more have sub-optimal levels.

There are a number of ways to get vitamin D, sun exposure being the most obvious one. Due to our modern lifestyle, however, most people don't get enough sun exposure and the vitamin D it provides. Supplementing vitamin D in pill form is an excellent alternative. 3,332 IU daily of vitamin D3 has been shown to sufficiently increase T levels by around 25%.[47] You can also get your vitamin D from seafoods such as salmon, mackerel, trout, cod liver oil, and tuna.

Magnesium: Magnesium is an essential mineral that aids in supporting the immune system, maintaining nerve and muscle function, and exerting a positive influence on the anabolic hormones. Typically, only 2% to 3% of T in the body is free. The aim is to have as much free T as possible. Magnesium assists with this goal by decreasing SHBG levels, allowing for more bio-available free T.

The recommended daily allowance for magnesium is 310 to 420 mg for healthy men. Magnesium can be found in foods such as green leafy vegetables, seeds, nuts, cocoa, and seafood. Spinach and salmon are also great sources of magnesium and contain the T booster's vitamin B and omega-3.

Zinc: Zinc is necessary for optimal T levels and other androgens. Low zinc levels can stop the pituitary gland from releasing the necessary hormones to stimulate T production. Even a moderate deficiency of zinc can produce negative effects. Men whose T level was less than 4.8 ng showed significant increases in T, sperm count, and DHT after taking zinc.[48] One study involving 40 men, between the ages of 20 to 80 years old, showed a significant correlation between zinc deficiency and decreased serum T.[49] When zinc supplementation was given to these marginally zinc-deficient men, there was an increase in T no matter the age.

Zinc containing foods include almonds, beef, baked beans, pumpkin seeds, eggs, liver, and certain seafood such as mollusks, salmon, and oysters. It's worth noting that zinc is excreted in sweat, so you may wish to supplement with zinc after a vigorous workout. It's recommended not to exceed more than 40 mg of zinc daily, which is the maximum dosage the body can safely tolerate.

While vitamin D, magnesium, and zinc are the crème de la crèm for optimal T, there are other secondary vitamins and minerals worth mentioning. They also have a role to play in regulating sex hormones and T production.

Vitamin A: There is a positive correlation between vitamin A and T production.[50] One of the ways vitamin A effects T production is by aiding in the absorption of fats. Ideally, a dietary fat intake of 35% or greater is needed for optimal T production. However, when there is a deficiency in vitamin A the body cannot efficiently utilize the dietary fats that are needed in T production.

Vitamin A is also used by the body to synthesize a plasma blood protein called transferrin glycoproteins. In addition to transporting iron into cells, transferrins transport cholesterol to the Leydig cells in the testicles. Once there the cholesterol is converted to T. Thus, a vitamin A deficiency directly correlates with impaired T production.

Vitamin A comes in two forms, preformed vitamin A and carotenoids. Preformed vitamin A comes from animal sources such as salmon, beef liver, and roasted chicken. Carotenoids can be found in plant sources such as carrots, sweet potatoes, and butternut squash. The daily recommended daily allowance of vitamin A for men is around 900 mcg.

Vitamin B: B vitamins each play a different role in T production. As previously mentioned, cholesterol is used as a precursor to T production. Vitamin B3 helps in this regard by regulating both good and bad cholesterol levels, which indirectly improves T. Foods that are rich in vitamin B3 include liver, chicken breast, tuna, turkey, salmon, anchovies, ground beef, avocados, peanuts, and brown rice, among others.

Vitamin B6 acts as a counterbalance for hormone regulation. When vitamin B6 is low, there's an increase in estrogen levels. As such, B6 suppresses the production of T-killing estrogen. Vitamin B6 foods include salmon, ricotta cheese, eggs, carrots, spinach, sweet potatoes, and bananas. Additionally, B6 can be found in the popular performance supplement ZMA which contains a blend of zinc, magnesium, and B6.

Finally there's vitamin B12 which aids in testicular health, sperm quality, and sperm count. A lack of B12 will correspond to a significant drop in T levels. Foods high in B12 are clams, sardines, trout, liver, fortified cereal, and salmon.

Vitamin C: Vitamin C may not be necessary for optimal T, but it can provide some indirect benefits. Vitamin C acts as a shield against oxidation, helping to protect T molecules. Additionally, vitamin C works to boost men's sperm count, quality, and motility. Since vitamin C is such a great antioxidant it also protects against the damaging effects of stress.

Vitamin E: Vitamin E was the fifth vitamin to be discovered in 1922, and aptly named after the fifth letter in the English alphabet. In the 1930s vitamin E was discovered to have antiestrogenic compounds and was used to treat infertility in both men and women. This was in part due to vitamin E's ability to alter estrogen and act as an anti-estrogen. Vitamin E, much like vitamin C, is a powerful antioxidant. These antioxidants work to fight against free radicals, protect against oxidative stress, and lowers polyunsaturated fats. Additionally, vitamin E helps to synthesize T, suppresses cortisol, and increase nitric oxide.

The effects of vitamin E were studied on both animals and humans in a 1982 Japanese study.[51] In the human part of the study, 11 healthy men between the ages of 30 and 69 were given a daily vitamin E dose of 483 mg. After eight weeks of vitamin E supplementation, their total T levels increased by an average of 30%, and their free T increased by 28%. The recommended daily allowance of vitamin E for males 15 and older is 15 mg (22 IU). Vitamin E can be found in the foods spinach, egg yolks, Brazil nuts, avocados, and shrimp.

Boron: Boron is a trace mineral that the body can't produce, but is commonly obtained from foods such as green leafy vegetables, coffee, apples, potatoes, beans, milk, raisins, and various types of nuts. Boron beneficially impacts the body's use of estrogen, T, vitamin D, and boosts magnesium absorption. Boron supplementation has demonstrated an increase in the levels of sex steroids in both men and women.

It was observed that after only one week of boron supplementation at 6 mg, there was a significant increase in free T and a significant decree in serum estradiol.[52] It was concluded that boron supplementation was particularly beneficial for aging men, whose SHBG levels increase with age while their free T declines with age.

When it comes to supplementation there is no specific daily recommended allowance. However, the Food and Nutrition Board of the Institute of Medicine recommends a daily upper limit dose of no more than 20 mg for adults aged 19 and up. Keep in mind that's the maximum daily amount. In reality, you really don't need much boron. Any more than 20 mg can be dangerous and produce unwanted side effects.

HERBS AND SUPPLEMENTS

There are some misconceptions concerning herbal supplements and about T boosters in general. There are those who believe that just because they don't produce the same effects as steroids they are somehow useless. It's true that if your T levels are already high and in optimal range they're not going to do much, but they are useful for those who have sub-optimal T levels. Since you're reading this book I assume this includes you. They are also useful for older individuals because as we get older SHBG increases and the androgen\estrogen ratio changes. Estrogen starts to become more dominant as we age. This is where herbs and supplements can help out.

There are a ton of herbs and supplements that claim to boost T, but there's not always the research available to back up those claims. Therefore, this chapter is divided into two parts. First, we'll look at the herbs and supplements that have studies verifying their claims. Then we'll look at herbs and supplements that "probably" don't work. I say probably because sometimes the research is not always conclusive. That's not to say that they don't provide other benefits, only that you shouldn't expect them to do much for your T levels.

Pine Pollen: As the name implies, pine pollen is the yellowish flour-like pollen found in pine cones. Pine pollen has been used in traditional Chinese medicine for thousands of years to restore health, increase longevity, and for its anti-aging properties. There's admittedly not a lot of research on pine pollen in regards to T. However, I've included it because it's the only known plant to contain androgenic substances including T, DHEA, androstenedione, and androsterone.

Pine pollen is generally considered safe but should be reserved for older men who have a mature endocrine system. Also, avoid pine pollen if you have any known pollen allergies.

Fenugreek: Fenugreek is an herb that's native to the Mediterranean region, southern Europe, and western Asia. The seeds are often used in cooking and for medicinal use. Many studies have found that fenugreek improves T levels, sexual performance, and libido. Males who took 300 mg of fenugreek twice daily in combination with resistance training demonstrated a steep increase in free T and a mild increase in total T.[53]

Testofen, a fenugreek extract, has also been shown to support free T, muscle mass, and libido in men. In one study of 60 healthy men, aged 25 to 52, demonstrated that Testofen was indeed beneficial. The study concluded that Testofen had significant positive effects on the physiological aspects of libido and may assist in maintaining healthy T levels.[54]

Longjack: Longjack, also known as Tongkat Ali and Pasak Bumi, is a root from the Eurycoma Longifolia green shrub tree, and native to Southeast Asia. It's commonly used to boost T levels and enhance the libido. Due to its ability to stimulate the production of androgen hormones, especially T, it has been used as a natural alternative to testosterone replacement therapy.[55] Both older men and women can also benefit from Longjack. 13 physically active seniors who were supplemented with 400 mg of Longjack daily for 5 weeks showed significant increases in total and free T as well as enhanced muscle strength.[56]

Stinging Nettle Root (SNR): SNR is a flowering plant that grows in Asia, Europe, Africa, and parts of North America. It gets its name from the stinging part of the plant, which can irritate the skin if touched. It's been found that the lignans in SNR prevent SHBG from binding with T, allowing more available free T.[57] Additionally, it works to inhibit aromatase activity, which prevents T from converting to estrogen. The most common dosage of SNR is 250 to 750 mg.

Ashwagandha: Also called Indian ginseng, ashwagandha is a small evergreen shrub found in India, the Middle East, and parts of Africa. Ashwagandha is an adaptogen that's commonly used for stress relief. In an 8-week placebo-controlled clinical study, 57 men between 18 and 50 were divided up into two groups. 29 subjects consumed 300 mg of ashwagandha root extract twice daily.[58] In comparison with the placebo group, the ashwagandha group showed significant increases in muscle strength, increased T levels, and a significant decrease in body fat percentage.

Ginger: Ginger has been shown to have many health benefits including lowering blood pressure, preventing cancers, and decreasing bad cholesterol. In regards to T, almost all the studies on ginger have been on animals. However, there is one study by Tikrit University on infertile men which showed a significant increase in sperm motility and count, as well as an 18% increase in T levels after treatment.[59]

Ginger is best taken in moderation. Too much ginger can cause sleepiness, thinning of the blood, heartburn, and low blood sugar levels, among others. For this reason, ginger should be avoided if you have hypoglycemia. Otherwise, 1 to 3 g is deemed sufficient.

Panax Ginseng: Panax ginseng is a root that's been used in Chinese medicine for thousands of years and provides many health benefits. Panax helps T both directly and indirectly. A clinical study on male fertility showed that Panax ginseng extract increased free T, total T, DHT, and several other hormones.[60] This was thanks to the chemical compounds found almost exclusively in Panax called ginsenosides.

Panax helps T indirectly by regulating blood glucose which in turn controls insulin levels. We have already noted the seesaw relationship between insulin and T. When one is up the other is down. Panax additionally increases nitric oxide which increases blood flow, improves libido, aids in building muscle mass, and boosts endurance. What's not to like about Panax? For supplementation use around 200 – 300 mg that is standardized to 20% – 30% ginsenosides.

Shilajit: Shilajit is a thick darkish substance found on rocks in the Himalayan Mountains formed by centuries of decomposing plants. It's commonly used in Indian Ayurvedic medicine for overall health and well-being. In one clinical study, healthy males between 45 and 55 were given a dose of 250 mg of purified Shilajit twice a day for 90 consecutive days. Subjects showed a significant increase in free T, total T, and DHEAS.[61]

When it comes to Shilajit quality is paramount as lesser quality can contain heavy metals. A purified organic form of Shilajit is preferred such as PrimaVie®. PrimaVie® is touted as the only Shilajit on the market to have GRAS approval (General Recognized as Safe by the FDA) and contains very low levels of heavy metals.

Saw Palmetto: Saw palmetto is a palm that's native to the southeastern United States, most commonly along the south Atlantic and Gulf coastal plains and sand hills. It's a very popular supplement for men for its purported ability to treat enlarged prostrates, prevent hair loss, and increase libido. Saw palmetto has also been linked to higher T levels. Researchers don't fully understand how saw palmetto works, only that it does. One possibility is that it slows down 5-alpha reductase, an enzyme that converts T into DHT, resulting in higher free T.

Diindolylmethane (DIM): If you recall, cruciferous vegetables contain a compound called indole-3-carbinol that converts to DIM and flushes estrogen from the body. The main difference between DIM and indole-3-carbinol is that DIM is the end product of metabolism. This makes DIM more stable since it requires no further conversion and breakdown by the stomach acids and provides immediate benefits.

Supplements That Probably Don't Work

Tribulus Terrestris (TT): TT is a plant found in the warm tropical regions of North America, Africa, Southern Eurasia, and Australia. It's a common ingredient in T boosting supplements, although the research doesn't support it. Eleven studies were looked at, including one patent application, to assess the effects of TT on both animals and humans. The data suggested that TT is ineffective for increasing T levels in humans.[62] The study concludes that "the nitric oxide release effect of TT may offer a plausible explanation for the observed physiological responses to TT supplementation, independent of the testosterone level."

Ginkgo Biloba: Ginkgo is a natural extract from the leaf of the Chinese Ginkgo tree. The Gingko tree is the oldest tree species on earth and it's been used in traditional Chinese medicine for thousands of years. In modern times it's used in alternative medicine to treat everything from anxiety to improving mental function.

Ginkgo is also a common ingredient in T boosting supplements, but the evidence is lacking. Studies indicate that it may raise T in rats, but humans are not rats. When put to the test, men and women who received 240 mg of Gingko daily for 14 days showed no significant changes to their T levels or other hormones.[63] There is, however, evidence to suggest that Ginkgo increases nitric oxide, which can help with erectile dysfunction in older men.[64]

Horny Goat Weed: As the name implies, horny goat weed is a well-known herb to improve sexual performance and boost libido. It's commonly used in many health supplements and T boosters. While it may be an effective aphrodisiac, there's no evidence to suggest that it helps increase T levels. All studies on horny goat weed have been on animals with mixed results. Some animal studies even showed a decrease in T levels and or an increase in estrogen when taken.

DHEA: DHEA is a naturally occurring steroid hormone produced by the adrenal glands as a precursor to male and female sex hormones, including T and estrogen. As a supplement, it's touted to improve sex drive, build muscle, and increase T. Studies on DHEA are mixed. Some smaller studies suggest DHEA can help stimulate T production, but just as many studies say the opposite. For instance, 28 men with low T were given a dose of 50 mg of DHEA twice daily and displayed no significant increase to their T levels.[65] Interestingly enough, several studies suggested DHEA may be more beneficial for women.

More studies are needed, but due to all the conflicting studies DHEA can't be recommended at this time to increase T. Additionally, DHEA can come with a host of side effects including but not limited to insomnia, high blood pressure, hair loss, and lowering good cholesterol. If DHEA is used long term or used excessively it could lead to even more serious problems such as Alzheimer-like symptoms, Cushing syndrome, and prostate cancer. If you still choose to use DHEA then do so sparingly.

Green Tea: Green tea is loaded with antioxidants and provides many health benefits. Unfortunately, when it comes to T the jury is still out. In theory, green tea contains an ingredient called epigallocatechin which inhibits the 5-alpha reductase enzyme. This then lessens the conversion of T into DHT, allowing for greater free T. The problem is there's no studies on humans to prove it yet. Studies on rats have shown that it does indeed increase T, but that may not translate to humans. Still, with so many health benefits of green tea, there's no reason not to drink it.

Maca: Known as Peruvian ginseng, Maca comes from the Andean region and is known as an aphrodisiac and fertility enhancer. Maca may provide many great benefits, but increasing T doesn't appear to be one of them. In one example, a 12-week study was conducted on healthy men between the ages of 21 and 56 years old.[66] They were given a dose of either 1500 mg or 3000 mg of Maca. The results showed no changes to their T levels or other selected hormones.

D-Aspartic Acid (DAA): DAA is a type of amino acid that works to produce and release hormones into the body. DAA is purported to increase T production in the brain and testicles. As a result, DAA is used in many T-boosting supplements. Most of the studies on DAA has been on animals rather than humans. The studies that are available on humans have yielded mixed results. Some studies have indicated that DAA increases T production, but other studies have not.

DAA may be of some benefit to men who have low T and are not physically active. However, DAA hasn't shown to be beneficial for men who are physically active. In fact, the opposite appears to be the case. Resistance trained males who were given 3 g of DAA showed no effects on their T markers. Those that were given 6 g daily actually showed a significant decrease in their free and total T levels.[67] Because resistance training plays such an important role in increasing and maintaining T levels, DAA cannot be fully endorsed.

Chrysin: Chrysin is a bioflavonoid commonly found in honey, propolis, mint, and blue passionflower. According to the FDA, chrysin is an aromatase inhibitor that prevents the conversion of T into estrogen and is used in treating high estrogen and low T. The problem is it has poor bioavailability. Only 1% actually gets absorbed by the body making it useless as a supplement. This further collaborates a study on male volunteers who were given chrysin rich foods consisting of honey and propolis over a 21-day period. They found that chrysin had no effect on the equilibrium of T in human males.[68]

TIPS FOR BETTER SLEEP

Sleep may not be the most interesting of topics, but it's on par with diet and exercise for optimizing T levels. As we sleep hormones are released into the bloodstream including HGH and insulin. Around 75% of HGH is released while we are asleep, which helps to build muscle, burn fat, increase libido and energy levels. Insulin is also released to remove glucose from the body to manage blood sugar levels.

If we don't get enough good quality sleep it adversely affects the hormones and chemicals in our bodies, which in turn negatively effects T levels. Just getting only 5 hours of sleep a night can lower T levels by as much as 10% to 15%, a condition that is common among 15% of the U.S. working population.[69] In the journal *Current Opinion of Endocrinology, Diabetes and Obesity*, Professor Gary Wittert says that getting enough sleep and at the right time is one of the most effective ways to raise T naturally.[70]

So how much sleep do we really need? The general consensus is 8 hours, give or take, of good quality sleep. Although this can vary from one individual to the other. Some people may need more or less sleep than others. Typically, younger individuals will require more sleep than older individuals. As Professor Wittert mentioned, the time you go to sleep is equally important. Ideally, you'll want to go to bed at around

10 p.m. and wake up around 6 a.m. for optimal hormonal balance.

Sleep is a deep subject with many books are dedicated solely to that topic alone. The goal of this chapter is not to give an in-depth discussion on sleep. Such a detailed analysis would go beyond the scope of this book. Instead, we'll look at a few key strategies to improve the quality of sleep and maximize your T levels.

Relax and unwind: Over the course of a 24-hour day, our brain frequencies will vary greatly. When we are awake our brain frequencies are high and are called beta waves (12 Hz to 40 Hz). When we are stressed or anxious they are at their highest and are called gamma waves (40 Hz to 100 Hz). As we relax and start to unwind they will slow down into alpha waves (8 Hz to 12 Hz). As we fall asleep they change into theta waves (4 Hz to 8 Hz). Finally, when we are in a deep sleep they are at their lowest and turn into delta waves (0 Hz to 4 Hz).

If your brain frequency is too high you won't be able to fall asleep or get good quality sleep. Therefore, start to relax and unwind one to two hours before bedtime. How you choose to unwind is largely up to you. For some, reading a book or writing in a journal is relaxing. For others, listening to soft music or taking a warm bath helps them to relax. Only you know what works best for you. Whatever you do make it a nightly routine and try to go to bed at the same time every night.

Magnesium: We've talked a lot about magnesium already. Yet another reason to love magnesium is for its ability to relax the muscles and reduce anxiety. Magnesium promotes deep restorative sleep by maintaining healthy levels of GABA, a neurotransmitter that promotes sleep. There are many types of magnesium available and some are better absorbed by the body than others. Magnesium citrate is the most recommended form of magnesium because it has a bioavailability of 90%, meaning it's easily absorbed by the body. One popular magnesium product on the market you might want to consider trying is Natural Vitality CALM.

Avoid blue light: Blue light emits a short wavelength that can delay the release of melatonin, increase alertness, and disrupt circadian rhythms making it more difficult to fall at sleep at night. Blue light can be found in fluorescent bulbs, LED lights, iPads, computer screens, TVs, smartphones, and other electronic devices.

Try avoiding all electronic devices that emit blue light an hour or two before bedtime. If that's not possible, or you would rather not, look into purchasing blue light blocking glasses. Conversely, there are several apps available that can filter out blue light during the evening and shift display colors to the warmer end of the spectrum. Macs and iPhones already have a feature called Night Shift that is built into their products for this express purpose.

Get sun in the morning: Light helps to regulate everything from our metabolism, body temperature, to sleep. That's why getting enough light, especially in the morning, helps to regulate sleep patterns. It's recommended to get 30 to 45 minutes of direct sunlight right after getting out of bed. That would be an ideal time for a morning walk if your schedule permits. Alternatively, you can purchase a lightbox that will mimic natural sunlight. Lightboxes tend to be expensive and don't put out as much light as natural sunlight. Still, they are an option for those who work the night shift or live in areas that don't receive much sunlight during the winter months.

Don't forget to exercise: Yet another reason to exercise is because it can help you sleep better. Studies have shown that exercise not only helps people to fall asleep more quickly but also improves the quality of their sleep. Even moderate aerobic activity for as little as 30 minutes has been shown helpful to induce sleep at bedtime. Also, contrary to popular belief, exercising at night hasn't been shown to negatively affect sleep quality.

Melatonin: Melatonin is a natural hormone in the body that controls the sleep-wake cycle. As it gets dark melatonin will increase in order to put you into a more restful state and promote sleep. Conversely, light exposure will cause the opposite effect and decrease melatonin levels. That's why it's best to dim the lights in the evening and avoid blue light to help the body prepare for sleep. For occasional difficulties sleeping, try taking 1 to 3 mg of melatonin two hours before bedtime.

Valerian root: Valerian root is a flowering plant native to Europe and Asia, but it can also be found in North America. It's often used for stress relief and in treating sleep and anxiety disorders. Studies have shown that valerian root can shorten the time it takes to fall asleep by as much as 15 to 20 minutes. However, it may take continuous use over several days for up to 4 weeks before the effects become noticeable. Valerian root is best when combined with other herbs, such as lemon balm. Take valerian root as directed 30 minutes to 2 hours before bedtime.

Chamomile: Chamomile comes from the name of several daisy-like plants of the Asteraceae family that's been used in traditional medicine for thousands of years. Chamomile contains an antioxidant called apigenin that binds to certain receptors in the brain to promote sleep. One study found that those who drank 270 mg of chamomile extract twice daily for 28 days decreased sleep latency by as much as 16 minutes.[71]

Avoid caffeine: Coffee, tea, and energy drinks are the most popular beverages for helping people to stay alert and boost energy. Everyone knows that caffeine is a stimulant, but not everyone knows just how long caffeine stays in their system. The physical effects of caffeine can be felt 45 minutes after consumption and has a half-life of around 5 hours. That means if you drink 40 mg of caffeine, then 5 hours later 20 mg is still in your system. However, it can take up to 10 hours for caffeine to completely clear from the system. It's best to avoid all caffeine products for 6 to 8 hours prior to bedtime so that it doesn't interfere with your sleep.

Avoid naps: It's not uncommon for people to take short naps when they have the opportunity to do so. For some taking a siesta is even part of their culture. But this can also make it more difficult to fall asleep at night. If this pertains to you then avoid napping. The longer you go without sleep the greater your sleep drive becomes. Also, avoid oversleeping in the morning as this too can make it difficult to fall asleep at night.

Insomnia: Perhaps you want a good night's sleep but for whatever reason, you can't seem to fall asleep. As someone who's struggled with insomnia, I know how frustrating that can be. There is, however, some strategies you can employ so that insomnia doesn't become chronic. If you're unable to fall asleep within 20 minutes, don't stay in bed. Lying in bed wide awake will only make you frustrated and further delay sleep. It can also create negative associations with your bed. Instead, get up for a while and read a book or listen to a podcast. Choose something that will not be too stimulating for your mind. Only when you feel tired should you go back to bed and try again.

Sometimes it seems no matter what you do, nothing seems to help. Everyone has trouble sleeping at some point in their lives. The key is not to focus on it. Go on about your day and don't worry if you didn't get a good night's sleep. When you start worrying and obsessing over sleep, that's when it can develop into a sleep disorder. Then you really have a problem.

Chronic insomnia is often the result of sleep anxiety and poor sleep hygiene. Sleep hygiene can be defined as the positive habits and practices that promote good sleep. The *American Academy of Sleep Medicine* recommends the following tips for better sleep, some of which we have already covered:[72]

- Keep a consistent sleep schedule. Get up at the same time every day, even on weekends or during vacations.
- Set a bedtime that is early enough for you to get at least 7 hours of sleep.
- Don't go to bed unless you are sleepy.
- If you don't fall asleep after 20 minutes, get out of bed.
- Establish a relaxing bedtime routine.
- Use your bed only for sleep and sex.
- Make your bedroom quiet and relaxing. Keep the room at a comfortable, cool temperature.
- Limit exposure to bright light in the evenings.

- Turn off electronic devices at least 30 minutes before bedtime.
- Don't eat a large meal before bedtime. If you are hungry at night, eat a light, healthy snack.
- Exercise regularly and maintain a healthy diet.
- Avoid consuming caffeine in the late afternoon or evening.
- Avoid consuming alcohol before bedtime.
- Reduce your fluid intake before bedtime.

STRESS MANAGEMENT

Stress is the body's natural physiological response to a threat or demand. Some degree of stress is natural and even healthy. It gives us the energy and focus to do the things we need to do. The problem is when we become too stressed for too long without sufficient time to recover. When the body is under stress, chemicals are flooded into the system. In particular, epinephrine (adrenaline), norepinephrine, and cortisol. Cortisol in particular adversely affects T levels. When cortisol goes up, T levels go down. Therefore, any strategies to optimize T levels should include stress management.

Stress can either be physical or psychological. When we are depressed, angry, or frustrated, it wears down on T levels over time. Even negative thoughts can produce stress. Stress reduction will require making positive lifestyle changes. If, for example, you work long hours, then strive to cut back on your hours if possible. Sometimes you may not be able to control every situation that causes stress, but you can control how you respond to stressful stimuli. This involves making a conscious decision to relax and let go of all the negative thoughts and emotions weighing you down. It will take time and practice for it to become natural and automatic.

Just remember that life's short, so strive to live a balanced life. Try to set aside at least 2 hours a day on things you enjoy doing rather it's working out, reading a book, or watching a good comedy. Laughter really is the best medicine and has been shown to reduce cortisol levels.[73] The following are additional tips and strategies to help you unwind and relax.

Relaxation Methods

Mindfulness Meditation: One effective tool for managing mental stress is with mindfulness meditation. Meditation is a process that involves focus, awareness, and relaxation. It works by activating the body's relaxation response via the HPA axis, the central stress response system. Mindfulness meditation is quite simple:

1. First, spend a few minutes getting comfortable.

2. Next, focus on your breathing by slowly inhaling and exhaling with your diaphragm.

3. Continue to focus on your breathing until relaxed.

The above is an example of a basic meditation exercise. If you're new to meditation you may find it challenging to stay focused, but this will improve with practice. If you find that meditation works for you, then consider studying mediation a little more in-depth. There are many great resources available on the topic. Many studies have verified the effectiveness of mediation for stress relief. Volunteers that participated in a four-day mindfulness meditation program showed a significant drop in their cortisol levels from 381.93 nmol/L to 306.38 nmol/L.[74]

The positive effects of deep abdominal breathing on stress have also been studied extensively and proven to be beneficial. In one study, 40 participants were divided into two groups, the breathing intervention group (BIG) and the control group (CG).[75] The BIG group received 20 intensive diaphragmatic breathing training sessions over 8 weeks, while the CG group did not. At the end of the study, the BIG group not only showed improved sustained attention levels but had a significant decrease in cortisol levels whereas the CG group did not.

Diaphragmatic breathing or abdominal breathing is fairly self-explanatory. Get yourself in a comfortable position and close your eyes. Focus on your breathing, inhaling slowly through your nose for 4 seconds. Remember to breathe through your abdomen and not your chest. Next, exhale slowly through pursed lips for 4 seconds. Repeat this exercise for 10 minutes or as desired. There are many types of breathing exercises and plenty of resources available on the internet. Choose the ones that work best for you.

Cognitive Behavioral Therapy (CBT): CBT is yet another tool for combating stress. Much of the stress we experience is due to negative thinking and behaviors. CBT works to change those negative thoughts and behaviors into positive ones. Not dwelling upon negative thoughts and feelings goes a long way towards accomplishing that. Better yet, challenge those negative thoughts by writing down evidence to the contrary. Journaling about your thoughts and feelings is a great way to overcome toxic thinking. CBT will require time and consistency to work, so don't expect change to happen overnight. It took time to accumulate stress, and it will take time to get rid of that stress. If ultimately you are unable to manage stress on your own consider talking with a therapist.

Yoga: Yoga is an excellent all-around stress reliever. A study was conducted to determine the effects of yoga on the psychological health of 90 individuals.[76] These 90 individuals were divided into two groups. One group practiced yoga for 8 weeks, while the other group practiced yoga for 16 weeks. The 8-week group did not start practicing yoga until the 8th week.

The study found significant reductions in stress and overall psychological health measures in both groups. The group that practiced yoga for 16 weeks showed significant decreases in stress, anxiety, and significant increases in well-being. Likewise, the group that practiced yoga for 8 weeks showed significant decreases in stress, anxiety, depression, and insomnia once they crossed over and started practicing yoga. Other such studies have yielded similar results.

Anti-Stress Vitamins & Minerals

Stress depletes the body of crucial vitamins and minerals. Deficiency in any of these vitamins and minerals make it harder for the body to counter the stress response, creating a vicious cycle. Try supplementing with the following vitamins and minerals to combat stress levels, reduce cortisol, and increase T levels.

Vitamins B & D: We've already seen how vitamin B and vitamin D work to optimize T production. As it happens, these vitamins are also great at combating against the effects of stress. Vitamins B6, B9, and B12 all have a number of positive effects on mood and stress.[77] Likewise, vitamin D significantly reduces cortisol levels by blocking a specific enzyme that is used in cortisol production.[78]

Vitamin C: The adrenal glands require vitamin C to make the necessary hormones to cope with stress and cortisol. The effects of vitamin C, along with vitamin B, were studied in 215 healthy males ranging in age from 30 to 55 years old.[79] The study concluded that supplementing a vitamin B complex with vitamin C led to improved ratings of stress. Additional benefits included better mental health, vigor, and improved cognitive performance during intense mental processing.

Potassium: Potassium is the third most abundant mineral in the body. Low levels of potassium have been linked to stress, anxiety, insomnia, and mental fatigue. Potassium supplementation helps to keep stress down and regulate blood pressure. It also helps muscles to relax in response to stress. Be aware that having too much potassium can cause unwanted side effects including numbness, nausea, and heart palpitations. Keep your potassium intake to 3,500 mg daily.

Magnesium: Magnesium promotes relaxation by binding to and stimulating gamma-aminobutyric acid (GABA) receptors in the brain. GABA is the primary neurotransmitter that slows down brain activity. When GABA is low, it can result in stress-related disorders such as anxiety. Additionally, magnesium restricts the release of stress hormones, including cortisol, by preventing them from entering the brain.

Zinc: One of the roles of zinc is to regulate stress hormones. It does this by blunting cortisol's release into the body and temporarily inhibiting cortisol secretion.[80] Zinc also helps to improve mood by regulating certain brain chemicals called neurotransmitters.

Calcium: Calcium acts as a natural sedative producing a calming, relaxing effect. Chronic stress depletes the body of calcium faster than it can be replaced by diet alone. When this happens, the body will seek homeostasis by leaching calcium from the bones and teeth, which can make them brittle over time. To prevent this, take calcium supplements along with vitamin D at mealtime for maximum absorption.

Anti-Stress Supplements

Ashwagandha: Ashwagandha isn't just a T booster; it also helps reduce cortisol levels. This was demonstrated in a double-blind, placebo-controlled study involving 64 subjects who had a history of chronic stress.[81] The treatment group took 300 mg of high-concentration full-spectrum ashwagandha extract twice daily for 60 days. Not only did the treatment group exhibit a significant reduction in scores on all the stress-assessment questionnaires, but they also showed a significant reduction in serum cortisol levels. The best form of Ashwagandha is KSM-66.

Ginger: This spice provides many health benefits, including fighting against the physical and psychological effects of stress. What makes ginger effective is the antioxidant gingerol, which helps to regulate cortisol production. Ginger is also an all-natural energy booster.

Ginkgo: Ginkgo may not do much your T levels, but it is useful for combating stress. Ginkgo works in two ways. The leaves contain a heavily oxidized terpene called ginkgolide that slows down the production of cortisol in the adrenal glands. Secondly, long term ginkgo use slows down the release of the hormone corticotropin that makes the adrenal gland produce cortisol. This was confirmed in a study of 70 healthy volunteers, which demonstrated ginkgo's ability to influence cortisol release in response to stress stimuli.[82]

Anti-Stress Food List

Garlic	Citrus Fruits	Raw Cacao
Bananas	Pears	Black or Green Tea
Holy Basil	Dried Apricots	Asparagus
Papaya	Kiwi	Pineapple
Kale	Avocados	Strawberries
Salmon	Brussel Sprouts	Blueberries
Red Bell Pepper	Broccoli	Green Leafy Vegetables
Grapefruit	Almonds	Cantaloupe
Yogurt	Tuna	Cauliflower
Potatoes	Spinach	Carrots
Cottage Cheese	Green Peas	Raspberries
Cherries	Brazil Nuts	Sweet Potatoes
Red Cabbage	Mushrooms	Tomatoes
Onions	Probiotic Foods	Mangos
Olive Oil	Cinnamon	Quinoa

7 SURPRISING THINGS THAT EFFECT TESTOSTERONE

Plastic Containers

Bisphenol A (BPA) is a chemical in plastics that can leech into our food and water supply. BPA has a negative effect on the endocrine system and alters T levels in men, estrogen, and sexual function. A study from China showed that men who worked around BPA in a chemical factory for six months had lower levels of T than men who worked in a tap water factory.[83] Plastics are all-pervasive and nearly impossible to eliminate completely. There are, however, things you can do to minimize your BPA exposure.

Ideally, the best solution is to eliminate bottled water completely. Instead, use glass containers and invest in a water filter, preferably one that is capable of reverse osmosis. Good quality water filters can be somewhat expensive, but they will pay for themselves in the long run. If you can't avoid bottled water totally, then at least pay attention to what they're made of. On every plastic bottle, usually on the bottom, there is a triangle with a number inside of it. This number indicates what the plastic is made of. The most toxic plastics that should be avoided are numbers #7, #3 and #6, while better options include numbers #1, #2, #4 and #5. Additionally, avoid microwaving food or liquids in plastic containers as this can cause BPA to leach into them more easily.

Need a BPA detox? Try sweating it out. One Canadian study found BPA in 16 of 20 participants tested.[84] Some of the subjects had BPA in their sweat but had no detectable BPA in their blood or urine samples. This study suggests that sweating is one way to eliminate BPA from the body. Besides working out, a sauna is another way to sweat BPA out of the body.

Environmental Factors

Believe it or not, our actions, thoughts, and even the environment around us can alter T levels. The reality is our T levels are always in flux throughout the day and change depending upon the situation. To illustrate this, an interesting experiment was conducted. A group of researchers from the University of Michigan at Ann Arbor hired actors to act out a scripted scene. In this scenario, an angry boss was scripted to fire a person from their job. The actors were encouraged to play an unfair boss who undermined and bullied their underling in the cruelest way possible. Saliva tests were taken both before and after the monologue was acted out. As you might have guessed, both the men and women showed elevated levels of T after acting out the scene.[85]

In another example of how environmental factors affect T levels, researchers from the Concordia University in Montreal recruited 39 young men in a study. Each one got to drive a very expensive Porsche 911 Carrera Cabriolet for one hour. They were then given an inexpensive 6-year-old Toyota Camry to drive around for one hour. Salvia tests revealed either no effect or a slight decline in T levels after they drove the Toyota Camry. However, there was a significant increase in T after driving the Porsche. Their hormones rose only slightly when they were driving on the open road with no spectators. The most significant increase came as they were driving around town with plenty of onlookers, especially of the female kind.[86]

Even having a dominating posture or talking to someone you find attractive can raise T levels. It's our reaction and perception of stimuli that alter T levels. The takeaway is we have a large degree of control over our T levels. Knowing this, always be mindful of how you respond to events as they occur. In every situation, strive to be confident, assertive, and bold, but do so in positive ways.

Truffle Aromatherapy

This may sound odd, but the scent of truffles, specifically black diamond truffles, has been linked to increased levels of T. That's right, you don't have to eat them you only need to smell them. It works the same way as aromatherapy does, through the process of olfaction.

The olfactory system is responsible for our sense of smell. When truffles are smelled, they send information to the brain that converts one kind of signal to another though a process known as transduction. The scent molecules reach the olfactory bulb and stimulate the hypothalamus gland, which in turn activates the pituitary gland to produce T.

This discovery was made by Dr. Moshe Shifrine, who noticed that when powdered truffle was added to pig feed in a very low dose, it increased weight gain and lean muscle. This is relevant because pigs are physiologically similar to humans, which is why they are often used in scientific research. Just the scent of the truffles alone was sufficient to increase T production. Dr. Shifrine sells his own truffle spray formula called Vitali-T-Boost.

Abstinence

It's commonly believed that having sex increases T production, but there's evidence to the contrary. It's true there will be a rise in T levels for a few hours after sexual activity. However, this is only temporary and has no lasting effects on T levels. In contrast, a study involving healthy men showed higher concentrations of T after a three-week abstinence break.[87] This was confirmed by a Chinese study involving 29 volunteers following periods of abstinence.[88]

The volunteer's serum T concentrations were examined daily during abstinence periods. There was not much change observed in their T levels from the 2nd to the 5th day of abstinence. However, on the 7th day, it increased by a whopping 145%. No regular fluctuations were observed after it peaked on the 7th day. This explains in part why male athletes will sometimes abstain from sexual activity prior to a major competition. The takeaway is that if you're really hardcore about raising T levels, then occasional abstinence breaks can be of some benefit.

Liver Health

The liver performs over 500 essential tasks including removing toxins from the body, protein synthesis, and producing digestive chemicals. Concerning T, the liver produces SHBG which binds to total T in order to regulate free T. The liver also produces a protein called albumin that binds to the remaining T. Unlike SHBG, however, albumin-bound T can easily be converted to free T. As a result, there's a direct correlation between liver health and T levels. This is further corroborated in a study involving men with advanced liver disease.

Men with cirrhosis of the liver were shown to have a 90% reduction in serum T levels.[89] Those levels continued to fall as their liver disease advanced. This means a healthy liver corresponds to healthy T levels. Lifestyle plays an important role in liver health. Limiting alcohol consumption, getting regular exercise, and eating a healthy diet all contribute to maintaining a healthy liver. Additionally, it's occasionally beneficial to detox the liver from time to time. Milk thistle, turmeric, and dandelion root are all good for cleansing the liver.

Watching Sports

As it turns out, men who watch sporting competitions can experience the same T surge as the players themselves, but only if their team wins. This is according to doctoral candidate Paul Bernhardt from the University of Utah. Bernhardt and his colleagues wanted to test the theory that fans who watched sporting events could have T changes similar to the athletes participating in the event.[90]

To prove this theory, Bernhardt and his team conducted two separate studies. In the first study, T was measured in male fans attending a basketball game. In the second study, T levels were measured among men who watched a soccer match. For the basketball study, researches collected saliva from 8 male spectators 1 hour before the game and 15 minutes after the game. For the soccer match, the researchers collected samples from 26 male spectators watching the event on television.

In both studies their T levels increased by as much as 20% in the fans of the winning teams. Unfortunately, fans of the losing team saw their T levels decrease by 20%. The researchers said, "The effect was likely sudden, rather than building up gradually during the game because the outcome was not determined until the last few seconds of each game." That makes another great reason to watch sports. Just hope your team wins!

Ambient Light

We've already established how sunlight is used to regulate circadian rhymes to enhance sleep, and it's also a good source of vitamin D. But sunlight can also raise T levels. It was previously observed that sexual interest varied with the seasons. It was postulated that ambient light may contribute to sexual desire. The scientists at the University of Siena in Italy set out to prove this hypothesis.[91]

They recruited 38 men who had a history with a lack of interest in sex. After an initial evaluation, they were divided into two groups. One group was treated with a specially adapted lightbox. The other placebo group was treated with a lightbox that was adapted to give out significantly less light. They were treated in the morning for 30 minutes daily for two weeks. Afterward, the scientists tested their sexual satisfaction and T levels.

The group that was treated with the full light treatment scored three times higher in sexual satisfaction compared to the placebo group that was exposed to lesser light. They also had an increase in T from an average of 2.1 ng/ml to 3.6 ng/ml whereas the placebo group showed no significant changes in T. Professor Andrea Fagiolini, the lead scientist, believes light therapy inhibits the pineal gland, which allows for the production of more T and causes other hormonal effects.

Incidentally, this was confirmed way back in 1939 by Abraham Myerson and Rudolph Neustadt at Boston State Hospital.[92] They measured the initial levels of circulating T in men and then exposed various parts of their bodies to UV light. Five days of chest exposure caused circulating T levels to increase by 120%. Eight days without UV exposure cause their T levels to return to initial levels. Oddly enough, when their genitals were exposed to UV light, T levels increased by 200%. So now you have a good excuse to join a nudist colony. Just kidding… mostly.

I hope you've found the information in this book useful. If so, please leave a rating and comment on Amazon. Thank you.

HIGH-T:
A Man's Guide for Boosting Testosterone

[1] Carlsen, E., Giwercman, A., Keiding, N., & Skakkebaek, N. E. (1992). Evidence for decreasing quality of semen during past 50 years. BMJ (Clinical research ed.), 305(6854), 609–613. https://doi.org/10.1136/bmj.305.6854.609

[2] Doheny, K. (2011, June 7). Testosterone Decline: Not Inevitable With Age? WebMD. https://www.webmd.com/healthy-aging/news/20110607/testosterone-decline-not-inevitable-with-age#1

[3] Paddock, C. (2012, June 25). Testosterone Does Not Necessarily Wane With Age. WebMD. https://www.medicalnewstoday.com/articles/247013

[4] Metzger, S. O., & Burnett, A. L. (2016). Impact of recent FDA ruling on testosterone replacement therapy (TRT). Translational andrology and urology, 5(6), 921–926. https://doi.org/10.21037/tau.2016.09.08

[5] MInguez-Alarcón, L., Chavarro, J. E., Mendiola, J., Roca, M., Tanrikut, C., Vioque, J., Jørgensen, N., & Torres-Cantero, A. M. (2017). Fatty acid intake in relation to reproductive hormones and testicular volume among young healthy men. Asian journal of andrology, 19(2), 184–190. https://doi.org/10.4103/1008-682X.190323

[6] Staff, S. X. (2009, June 14). Testosterone Decreases after Ingestion of Sugar. Testosterone Decreases after Ingestion of Sugar. https://medicalxpress.com/news/2009-06-testosterone-decreases-ingestion-sugar.html

[7] Röjdmark, S., Asplund, A., & Rössner, S. (1989). Pituitary-testicular axis in obese men during short-term fasting. Acta endocrinologica, 121(5), 727–732. https://doi.org/10.1530/acta.0.1210727

[8] Ho, K. Y., Veldhuis, J. D., Johnson, M. L., Furlanetto, R., Evans, W. S., Alberti, K. G., & Thorner, M. O. (1988). Fasting enhances growth hormone secretion and amplifies the complex rhythms of growth

hormone secretion in man. The Journal of clinical investigation, 81(4), 968–975. https://doi.org/10.1172/JCI113450

[9] C. Longcope, H. A. Feldman, J. B. McKinlay, A. B. Araujo, Diet and Sex Hormone-Binding Globulin, The Journal of Clinical Endocrinology & Metabolism, Volume 85, Issue 1, 1 January 2000, Pages 293–296, https://doi.org/10.1210/jcem.85.1.6291

[10] Dorgan, J. F., Judd, J. T., Longcope, C., Brown, C., Schatzkin, A., Clevidence, B. A., Campbell, W. S., Nair, P. P., Franz, C., Kahle, L., & Taylor, P. R. (1996). Effects of dietary fat and fiber on plasma and urine androgens and estrogens in men: a controlled feeding study. The American journal of clinical nutrition, 64(6), 850–855. https://doi.org/10.1093/ajcn/64.6.850

[11] Sallinen, Janne & Pakarinen, A & Ahtiainen, Juha & Kraemer, William & Volek, J & Häkkinen, Keijo. (2004). Relationship Between Diet and Serum Anabolic Hormone Responses to Heavy-Resistance Exercise in Men. International journal of sports medicine. 25. 627-33. 10.1055/s-2004-815818.

[12] Hämäläinen, E., Adlercreutz, H., Puska, P., & Pietinen, P. (1984). Diet and serum sex hormones in healthy men. Journal of steroid biochemistry, 20(1), 459–464. https://doi.org/10.1016/0022-4731(84)90254-1

[13] Christina Wang, Don H. Catlin, Borislav Starcevic, David Heber, Christie Ambler, Nancy Berman, Geraldine Lucas, Andrew Leung, Kathy Schramm, Paul W. N. Lee, Laura Hull, Ronald S. Swerdloff, Low-Fat High-Fiber Diet Decreased Serum and Urine Androgens in Men, The Journal of Clinical Endocrinology & Metabolism, Volume 90, Issue 6, 1 June 2005, Pages 3550–3559, https://doi.org/10.1210/jc.2004-1530

[14] Derouiche, A., Jafri, A., Driouch, I., El Khasmi, M., Adlouni, A., Benajiba, N., Bamou, Y., Saile, R., & Benouhoud, M. (2013). Effect of argan and olive oil consumption on the hormonal profile of androgens among healthy adult Moroccan men. Natural product communications, 8(1), 51–53.

[15] Hu FB, Stampfer MJ, Rimm EB, et al. A Prospective Study of Egg Consumption and Risk of Cardiovascular Disease in Men and

Women. JAMA. 1999;281(15):1387–1394. doi:10.1001/jama.281.15.1387

[16] DiMarco, D. M., Missimer, A., Murillo, A. G., Lemos, B. S., Malysheva, O. V., Caudill, M. A., Blesso, C. N., & Fernandez, M. L. (2017). Intake of up to 3 Eggs/Day Increases HDL Cholesterol and Plasma Choline While Plasma Trimethylamine-N-oxide is Unchanged in a Healthy Population. Lipids, 52(3), 255–263. https://doi.org/10.1007/s11745-017-4230-9

[17] Heller, R. F., Wheeler, M. J., Micallef, J., Miller, N. E., & Lewis, B. (1983). Relationship of high density lipoprotein cholesterol with total and free testosterone and sex hormone binding globulin. Acta endocrinologica, 104(2), 253–256. https://doi.org/10.1530/acta.0.1040253

[18] Grube BJ, Eng ET, Kao YC, Kwon A, Chen S. White button mushroom phytochemicals inhibit aromatase activity and breast cancer cell proliferation. J Nutr. 2001;131(12):3288-3293. doi:10.1093/jn/131.12.3288

[19] Pizzorno L. (2015). Nothing Boring About Boron. Integrative medicine (Encinitas, Calif.), 14(4), 35–48.

[20] Shing, C. M., Chong, S., Driller, M. W., & Fell, J. W. (2016). Acute protease supplementation effects on muscle damage and recovery across consecutive days of cycle racing. European journal of sport science, 16(2), 206–212. https://doi.org/10.1080/17461391.2014.1001878

[21] Wang, Y., Lee, K. W., Chan, F. L., Chen, S., & Leung, L. K. (2006). The red wine polyphenol resveratrol displays bilevel inhibition on aromatase in breast cancer cells. Toxicological sciences : an official journal of the Society of Toxicology, 92(1), 71–77. https://doi.org/10.1093/toxsci/kfj190

[22] Topo, E., Soricelli, A., D'Aniello, A., Ronsini, S., & D'Aniello, G. (2009). The role and molecular mechanism of D-aspartic acid in the release and synthesis of LH and testosterone in humans and rats. Reproductive biology and endocrinology : RB&E, 7, 120. https://doi.org/10.1186/1477-7827-7-120

[23] Mero, A., Pitkänen, H., Oja, S. S., Komi, P. V., Pöntinen, P., & Takala, T. (1997). Leucine supplementation and serum amino acids,

testosterone, cortisol and growth hormone in male power athletes during training. The Journal of sports medicine and physical fitness, 37(2), 137–145.

[24] Sierksma, A., Sarkola, T., Eriksson, C. J., van der Gaag, M. S., Grobbee, D. E., & Hendriks, H. F. (2004). Effect of moderate alcohol consumption on plasma dehydroepiandrosterone sulfate, testosterone, and estradiol levels in middle-aged men and postmenopausal women: a diet-controlled intervention study. Alcoholism, clinical and experimental research, 28(5), 780–785. https://doi.org/10.1097/01.alc.0000125356.70824.81

[25] Frias, J., Torres, J. M., Miranda, M. T., Ruiz, E., & Ortega, E. (2002). Effects of acute alcohol intoxication on pituitary-gonadal axis hormones, pituitary-adrenal axis hormones, beta-endorphin and prolactin in human adults of both sexes. Alcohol and alcoholism (Oxford, Oxfordshire), 37(2), 169–173. https://doi.org/10.1093/alcalc/37.2.169

[26] Glenn Braunstein and James Klinenberg. (2008) Environmental Gynecomastia. Endocrine Practice 14:4, 409-411. Online publication date: 16-Jun-2008.

[27] Dillingham, B. L., McVeigh, B. L., Lampe, J. W., & Duncan, A. M. (2005). Soy protein isolates of varying isoflavone content exert minor effects on serum reproductive hormones in healthy young men. The Journal of nutrition, 135(3), 584–591. https://doi.org/10.1093/jn/135.3.584

[28] Chavarro, J. E., Toth, T. L., Sadio, S. M., & Hauser, R. (2008). Soy food and isoflavone intake in relation to semen quality parameters among men from an infertility clinic. Human reproduction (Oxford, England), 23(11), 2584–2590. https://doi.org/10.1093/humrep/den243

[29] Hamilton-Reeves, J. M., Vazquez, G., Duval, S. J., Phipps, W. R., Kurzer, M. S., & Messina, M. J. (2010). Clinical studies show no effects of soy protein or isoflavones on reproductive hormones in men: results of a meta-analysis. Fertility and sterility, 94(3), 997–1007. https://doi.org/10.1016/j.fertnstert.2009.04.038

[30] Clair, E., Mesnage, R., Travert, C., & Séralini, G. É. (2012). A glyphosate-based herbicide induces necrosis and apoptosis in

mature rat testicular cells in vitro, and testosterone decrease at lower levels. Toxicology in vitro : an international journal published in association with BIBRA, 26(2), 269–279. https://doi.org/10.1016/j.tiv.2011.12.009

[31] Thompson LU. In: Flaxseed in Human Nutrition. Cunnane SC and Thompson LU, eds. Champaign, IL: AOCS Press, 1995, pp. 219-236.

[32] Maruyama, K., Oshima, T., & Ohyama, K. (2010). Exposure to exogenous estrogen through intake of commercial milk produced from pregnant cows. Pediatrics international : official journal of the Japan Pediatric Society, 52(1), 33–38. https://doi.org/10.1111/j.1442-200X.2009.02890.x

[33] Ganmaa, Davaasambuu & Wang, Peiyu & Qin, L.Q. & Hoshi, K & Sato, A. (2001). Is milk repossible for male reproductive disorders. Medical hypotheses. 57. 510-4. 10.1054/mehy.2001.1380.

[34] Malekinejad, H., & Rezabakhsh, A. (2015). Hormones in Dairy Foods and Their Impact on Public Health - A Narrative Review Article. Iranian journal of public health, 44(6), 742–758.

[35] Armanini, D., Bonanni, G., Mattarello, M. J., Fiore, C., Sartorato, P., & Palermo, M. (2003). Licorice consumption and serum testosterone in healthy man. Experimental and clinical endocrinology & diabetes : official journal, German Society of Endocrinology [and] German Diabetes Association, 111(6), 341–343. https://doi.org/10.1055/s-2003-42724

[36] Estrogenic and Antiproliferative Properties of Glabridin from Licorice in Human Breast Cancer Cells
Snait Tamir, Mark Eizenberg, Dalia Somjen, Naftali Stern, Rayah Shelach, Alvin Kaye and Jacob Vaya
Cancer Res October 15 2000 (60) (20) 5704-5709;

[37] Omar, H. R., Komarova, I., El-Ghonemi, M., Fathy, A., Rashad, R., Abdelmalak, H. D., Yerramadha, M. R., Ali, Y., Helal, E., & Camporesi, E. M. (2012). Licorice abuse: time to send a warning message. Therapeutic advances in endocrinology and metabolism, 3(4), 125–138. https://doi.org/10.1177/2042018812454322

[38] Kalgaonkar, S., Almario, R., Gurusinghe, D. et al. Differential effects of walnuts vs almonds on improving metabolic and

endocrine parameters in PCOS. Eur J Clin Nutr 65, 386–393 (2011). https://doi.org/10.1038/ejcn.2010.266

[39] Boué, S. M., Wiese, T. E., Nehls, S., Burow, M. E., Elliott, S., Carter-Wientjes, C. H., Shih, B. Y., McLachlan, J. A., & Cleveland, T. E. (2003). Evaluation of the estrogenic effects of legume extracts containing phytoestrogens. Journal of agricultural and food chemistry, 51(8), 2193–2199. https://doi.org/10.1021/jf021114s

[40] Simopoulos A. P. (2002). The importance of the ratio of omega-6/omega-3 essential fatty acids. Biomedicine & pharmacotherapy = Biomedecine & pharmacotherapie, 56(8), 365–379. https://doi.org/10.1016/s0753-3322(02)00253-6

[41] Craig, B. W., Brown, R., & Everhart, J. (1989). Effects of progressive resistance training on growth hormone and testosterone levels in young and elderly subjects. Mechanisms of ageing and development, 49(2), 159–169. https://doi.org/10.1016/0047-6374(89)90099-7

[42] Shaner, A. A., Vingren, J. L., Hatfield, D. L., Budnar, R. G., Jr, Duplanty, A. A., & Hill, D. W. (2014). The acute hormonal response to free weight and machine weight resistance exercise. Journal of strength and conditioning research, 28(4), 1032–1040. https://doi.org/10.1519/JSC.0000000000000317

[43] Cook, C., Beaven, C. M., Kilduff, L. P., & Drawer, S. (2012). Acute caffeine ingestion's increase of voluntarily chosen resistance-training load after limited sleep. International journal of sport nutrition and exercise metabolism, 22(3), 157–164. https://doi.org/10.1123/ijsnem.22.3.157

[44] Paton, Carl & Hopkins, Will & Cook, Christian. (2009). Effects of Low- vs. High-Cadence Interval Training on Cycling Performance. Journal of strength and conditioning research / National Strength & Conditioning Association. 23. 1758-63. 10.1519/JSC.0b013e3181b3f1d3.

[45] Stokes, K. A., Nevill, M. E., Hall, G. M., & Lakomy, H. K. (2002). The time course of the human growth hormone response to a 6 s and a 30 s cycle ergometer sprint. Journal of sports sciences, 20(6), 487–494. https://doi.org/10.1080/02640410252925152

[46] Wehr, E., Pilz, S., Boehm, B. O., März, W., & Obermayer-Pietsch, B. (2010). Association of vitamin D status with serum androgen levels in men. Clinical endocrinology, 73(2), 243–248. https://doi.org/10.1111/j.1365-2265.2009.03777.x

[47] Pilz, S., Frisch, S., Koertke, H., Kuhn, J., Dreier, J., Obermayer-Pietsch, B., Wehr, E., & Zittermann, A. (2011). Effect of vitamin D supplementation on testosterone levels in men. Hormone and metabolic research = Hormon- und Stoffwechselforschung = Hormones et metabolisme, 43(3), 223–225. https://doi.org/10.1055/s-0030-1269854

[48] Netter, A., Hartoma, R., & Nahoul, K. (1981). Effect of zinc administration on plasma testosterone, dihydrotestosterone, and sperm count. Archives of andrology, 7(1), 69–73. https://doi.org/10.3109/01485018109009378

[49] Prasad, A. S., Mantzoros, C. S., Beck, F. W., Hess, J. W., & Brewer, G. J. (1996). Zinc status and serum testosterone levels of healthy adults. Nutrition (Burbank, Los Angeles County, Calif.), 12(5), 344–348. https://doi.org/10.1016/s0899-9007(96)80058-x

[50] Bishop, D. T., Meikle, A. W., Slattery, M. L., Stringham, J. D., Ford, M. H., & West, D. W. (1988). The effect of nutritional factors on sex hormone levels in male twins. Genetic epidemiology, 5(1), 43–59. https://doi.org/10.1002/gepi.1370050105

[51] Umeda, F., Kato, K., Muta, K., & Ibayashi, H. (1982). Effect of vitamin E on function of pituitary-gonadal axis in male rats and human subjects. Endocrinologia japonica, 29(3), 287–292. https://doi.org/10.1507/endocrj1954.29.287

[52] Pizzorno L. (2015). Nothing Boring About Boron. Integrative medicine (Encinitas, Calif.), 14(4), 35–48.

[53] Wankhede, S., Mohan, V., & Thakurdesai, P. (2016). Beneficial effects of fenugreek glycoside supplementation in male subjects during resistance training: A randomized controlled pilot study. Journal of sport and health science, 5(2), 176–182. https://doi.org/10.1016/j.jshs.2014.09.005

[54] Steels, E., Rao, A., & Vitetta, L. (2011). Physiological aspects of male libido enhanced by standardized Trigonella foenum-graecum

extract and mineral formulation. Phytotherapy research : PTR, 25(9), 1294–1300. https://doi.org/10.1002/ptr.3360
[55] Mohd Effendy, N., Mohamed, N., Muhammad, N., Naina Mohamad, I., & Shuid, A. N. (2012). Eurycoma longifolia: Medicinal Plant in the Prevention and Treatment of Male Osteoporosis due to Androgen Deficiency. Evidence-based complementary and alternative medicine : eCAM, 2012, 125761. https://doi.org/10.1155/2012/125761
[56] Henkel, R. R., Wang, R., Bassett, S. H., Chen, T., Liu, N., Zhu, Y., & Tambi, M. I. (2014). Tongkat Ali as a potential herbal supplement for physically active male and female seniors--a pilot study. Phytotherapy research : PTR, 28(4), 544–550. https://doi.org/10.1002/ptr.5017
[57] Schöttner, M., Gansser, D., & Spiteller, G. (1997). Lignans from the roots of Urtica dioica and their metabolites bind to human sex hormone binding globulin (SHBG). Planta medica, 63(6), 529–532. https://doi.org/10.1055/s-2006-957756
[58] Wankhede, S., Langade, D., Joshi, K. et al. Examining the effect of Withania somnifera supplementation on muscle strength and recovery: a randomized controlled trial. J Int Soc Sports Nutr 12, 43 (2015). https://doi.org/10.1186/s12970-015-0104-9
[59] Mares AK, Abid W, Najam WS. The effect of Ginger on semen parameters and serum FSH, LH & testosterone of infertile men. Tikrit Med J. 2012;18:322.
[60] Salvati, G., Genovesi, G., Marcellini, L., Paolini, P., De Nuccio, I., Pepe, M., & Re, M. (1996). Effects of Panax Ginseng C.A. Meyer saponins on male fertility. Panminerva medica, 38(4), 249–254.
[61] Pandit, S., Biswas, S., Jana, U., De, R. K., Mukhopadhyay, S. C., & Biswas, T. K. (2016). Clinical evaluation of purified Shilajit on testosterone levels in healthy volunteers. Andrologia, 48(5), 570–575. https://doi.org/10.1111/and.12482
[62] Qureshi, A., Naughton, D. P., & Petroczi, A. (2014). A systematic review on the herbal extract Tribulus terrestris and the roots of its putative aphrodisiac and performance enhancing effect. Journal of dietary supplements, 11(1), 64–79. https://doi.org/10.3109/19390211.2014.887602

[63] Markowitz, J. S., DeVane, C. L., Lewis, J. G., Chavin, K. D., Wang, J. S., & Donovan, J. L. (2005). Effect of Ginkgo biloba extract on plasma steroid concentrations in healthy volunteers: a pilot study. Pharmacotherapy, 25(10), 1337–1340. https://doi.org/10.1592/phco.2005.25.10.1337

[64] McKay D. (2004). Nutrients and botanicals for erectile dysfunction: examining the evidence. Alternative medicine review : a journal of clinical therapeutic, 9(1), 4–16.

[65] Morales, A., Black, A., Emerson, L., Barkin, J., Kuzmarov, I., & Day, A. (2009). Androgens and sexual function: a placebo-controlled, randomized, double-blind study of testosterone vs. dehydroepiandrosterone in men with sexual dysfunction and androgen deficiency. The aging male : the official journal of the International Society for the Study of the Aging Male, 12(4), 104–112. https://doi.org/10.3109/13685530903294388

[66] Gonzales, G. F., Córdova, A., Vega, K., Chung, A., Villena, A., & Góñez, C. (2003). Effect of Lepidium meyenii (Maca), a root with aphrodisiac and fertility-enhancing properties, on serum reproductive hormone levels in adult healthy men. The Journal of endocrinology, 176(1), 163–168. https://doi.org/10.1677/joe.0.1760163

[67] Melville, G. W., Siegler, J. C., & Marshall, P. W. (2015). Three and six grams supplementation of d-aspartic acid in resistance trained men. Journal of the International Society of Sports Nutrition, 12, 15. https://doi.org/10.1186/s12970-015-0078-7

[68] Gambelunghe, C., Rossi, R., Sommavilla, M., Ferranti, C., Rossi, R., Ciculi, C., Gizzi, S., Micheletti, A., & Rufini, S. (2003). Effects of chrysin on urinary testosterone levels in human males. Journal of medicinal food, 6(4), 387–390. https://doi.org/10.1089/109662003772519967

[69] Leproult R, Van Cauter E. Effect of 1 Week of Sleep Restriction on Testosterone Levels in Young Healthy Men. JAMA. 2011;305(21):2173–2174. doi:10.1001/jama.2011.710

[70] Wittert G. (2014). The relationship between sleep disorders and testosterone. Current opinion in endocrinology, diabetes, and

obesity, 21(3), 239–243. https://doi.org/10.1097/MED.0000000000000069

[71] Zick, S. M., Wright, B. D., Sen, A., & Arnedt, J. T. (2011). Preliminary examination of the efficacy and safety of a standardized chamomile extract for chronic primary insomnia: a randomized placebo-controlled pilot study. BMC complementary and alternative medicine, 11, 78. https://doi.org/10.1186/1472-6882-11-78

[72] Healthy Sleep Habits and Good Sleep Hygiene. (n.d.). Http://Sleepeducation.Org/Essentials-in-Sleep/Healthy-Sleep-Habits. Retrieved August 1, 2020, from http.//sleepeducation.org/essentials-in-sleep/healthy-sleep-habits

[73] Berk, L. S., Tan, S. A., Fry, W. F., Napier, B. J., Lee, J. W., Hubbard, R. W., Lewis, J. E., & Eby, W. C. (1989). Neuroendocrine and stress hormone changes during mirthful laughter. The American journal of the medical sciences, 298(6), 390–396. https://doi.org/10.1097/00000441-198912000-00006

[74] Turakitwanakan, W., Mekseepralard, C., & Busarakumtragul, P. (2013). Effects of mindfulness meditation on serum cortisol of medical students. Journal of the Medical Association of Thailand = Chotmaihet thangphaet, 96 Suppl 1, S90–S95.

[75] Ma, X., Yue, Z. Q., Gong, Z. Q., Zhang, H., Duan, N. Y., Shi, Y. T., Wei, G. X., & Li, Y. F. (2017). The Effect of Diaphragmatic Breathing on Attention, Negative Affect and Stress in Healthy Adults. Frontiers in psychology, 8, 874. https://doi.org/10.3389/fpsyg.2017.00874

[76] Maddux, R. E., Daukantaité, D., & Tellhed, U. (2018). The effects of yoga on stress and psychological health among employees: an 8- and 16-week intervention study. Anxiety, stress, and coping, 31(2), 121–134. https://doi.org/10.1080/10615806.2017.1405261

[77] Camfield, D. A., Wetherell, M. A., Scholey, A. B., Cox, K. H., Fogg, E., White, D. J., Sarris, J., Kras, M., Stough, C., Sali, A., & Pipingas, A. (2013). The effects of multivitamin supplementation on diurnal cortisol secretion and perceived stress. Nutrients, 5(11), 4429–4450. https://doi.org/10.3390/nu5114429

[78] Al-Dujaili, E. A., Munir, N., & Iniesta, R. R. (2016). Effect of vitamin D supplementation on cardiovascular disease risk factors and exercise performance in healthy participants: a randomized placebo-controlled preliminary study. Therapeutic advances in endocrinology and metabolism, 7(4), 153–165. https://doi.org/10.1177/2042018816653357

[79] Kennedy, D. O., Veasey, R., Watson, A., Dodd, F., Jones, E., Maggini, S., & Haskell, C. F. (2010). Effects of high-dose B vitamin complex with vitamin C and minerals on subjective mood and performance in healthy males. Psychopharmacology, 211(1), 55–68. https://doi.org/10.1007/s00213-010-1870-3

[80] Brandão-Neto, J., de Mendonça, B. B., Shuhama, T., Marchini, J. S., Pimenta, W. P., & Tornero, M. T. (1990). Zinc acutely and temporarily inhibits adrenal cortisol secretion in humans. A preliminary report. Biological trace element research, 24(1), 83–89. https://doi.org/10.1007/BF02789143

[81] Chandrasekhar, K., Kapoor, J., & Anishetty, S. (2012). A prospective, randomized double-blind, placebo-controlled study of safety and efficacy of a high-concentration full-spectrum extract of ashwagandha root in reducing stress and anxiety in adults. Indian journal of psychological medicine, 34(3), 255–262. https://doi.org/10.4103/0253-7176.106022

[82] Jezova, D., Duncko, R., Lassanova, M., Kriska, M., & Moncek, F. (2002). Reduction of rise in blood pressure and cortisol release during stress by Ginkgo biloba extract (EGb 761) in healthy volunteers. Journal of physiology and pharmacology : an official journal of the Polish Physiological Society, 53(3), 337–348.

[83] Rettner, R. (2013, May 8). BPA Linked with Lower Testosterone. Live Science. https://www.livescience.com/29401-bpa-testosterone-levels.html

[84] Genuis, S. J., Beesoon, S., Birkholz, D., & Lobo, R. A. (2012). Human excretion of bisphenol A: blood, urine, and sweat (BUS) study. Journal of environmental and public health, 2012, 185731. https://doi.org/10.1155/2012/185731

[85] Newitz, A. (2015, November 5). You Can Raise Your Testosterone Levels Just By Acting Aggressive. Gizmodo.

https://gizmodo.com/you-can-raise-your-testosterone-levels-just-by-acting-a-1740178167

[86] Hagan, P. (2009, October 13). Fast cars boost men's testosterone levels: research. The Telegraph. https://www.telegraph.co.uk/news/health/news/6316522/Fast-cars-boost-mens-testosterone-levels-research.html

[87] Exton, M. S., Krüger, T. H., Bursch, N., Haake, P., Knapp, W., Schedlowski, M., & Hartmann, U. (2001). Endocrine response to masturbation-induced orgasm in healthy men following a 3-week sexual abstinence. World journal of urology, 19(5), 377–382. https://doi.org/10.1007/s003450100222

[88] Jiang, M., Xin, J., Zou, Q., & Shen, J. W. (2003). A research on the relationship between ejaculation and serum testosterone level in men. Journal of Zhejiang University. Science, 4(2), 236–240. https://doi.org/10.1631/jzus.2003.0236

[89] Sinclair, M., Grossmann, M., Gow, P. J., & Angus, P. W. (2015). Testosterone in men with advanced liver disease: abnormalities and implications. Journal of gastroenterology and hepatology, 30(2), 244–251. https://doi.org/10.1111/jgh.12695

[90] Bernhardt, P. C., Dabbs, J. M., Jr, Fielden, J. A., & Lutter, C. D. (1998). Testosterone changes during vicarious experiences of winning and losing among fans at sporting events. Physiology & behavior, 65(1), 59–62. https://doi.org/10.1016/s0031-9384(98)00147-4

[91] European College of Neuropsychopharmacology (ECNP). (2016, September 18). Lack of interest in sex successfully treated by exposure to bright light. ScienceDaily. Retrieved August 4, 2020 from www.sciencedaily.com/releases/2016/09/160918214443.htm

[92] ABRAHAM MYERSON, RUDOLPH NEUSTADT, INFLUENCE OF ULTRAVIOLET IRRADIATION UPON EXCRETION OF SEX HORMONES IN THE MALE1, Endocrinology, Volume 25, Issue 1, 1 July 1939, Pages 7–12, https://doi.org/10.1210/endo-25-1-7

Made in the USA
Las Vegas, NV
27 March 2025